What People Are Saying About

Adventures of an American Medical Student

Adventures of an American Medical Student gives a first-hand look into what medical students in the United States go through in their medical education. It is a very candid story about one medical student's events throughout his medical education journey. The stories are captivating and keep the reader wanting to read more. I can relate to some of the stories from when I was a medical student. The stress, long work hours, interesting patient stories, and the balance of school and personal life are vividly illustrated in this book. For anyone wanting to know what a day in the life of a medical student looks like, this helps demonstrate that from one day to the next.

—Joe Kingery, D.O.
Dean, Kentucky College of Osteopathic Medicine
Professor of Family Medicine

Dr. Champion pulls the curtain back on medical training with his first novel. He effectively captures the contrast between the mind-numbing monotony and unfiltered chaos that is the second half of medical school. Thought provoking and honest throughout, *Adventures of an American Medical Student* tells an endearing story that few outside the field would ever get to experience.

—Matthew DeLiere, M.D.
Forensic Psychiatrist
Denver, Colorado

This book invited me to relive my own medical school training, both the glory and the misery. It will give the non-medical reader a realistic and fascinating look into the medical training process and how it impacts both the medical office and the student's personal life.

—**C. Allen Musil, M.D.**

Medical Director, Frontier Health

Chair, East Tennessee State University Department of Psychiatry

JC has effectively combined his medical school clinical years with entertainment and crisp medical review. A seasoned physician will appreciate a refreshing review, while any medical student or resident will anticipate and seek similar experiences.

—**Richard Hilliard, D.O.**

Internist

Major, U.S. Army, retired

Adventures of an American Medical Student

Adventures of an American Medical Student

By James Champion

ROUNDFIRE
BOOKS

Winchester, UK
Washington, USA

JOHN HUNT PUBLISHING

First published by Roundfire Books, 2024
Roundfire Books is an imprint of John Hunt Publishing Ltd., No. 3 East St., Alresford,
Hampshire SO24 9EE, UK
office@jhpbooks.com
www.johnhuntpublishing.com
www.roundfire-books.com

For distributor details and how to order please visit the 'Ordering' section on our website.

Text copyright: James Champion 2023

ISBN: 978 1 80341 498 0
978 1 80341 499 7 (ebook)
Library of Congress Control Number: 2023900932

A CIP catalogue record for this book is available from the British Library.

Design: Lapiz Digital Services

UK: Printed and bound by CPI Group (UK) Ltd, Croydon, CR0 4YY
Printed in North America by CPI GPS partners

We operate a distinctive and ethical publishing philosophy in
all areas of our business, from our global network of authors to
production and worldwide distribution.

In memory of my mother, Carol. She was an angel on Earth.

Medicine is a severe mistress.
—Kenneth Akers, D.O.
Hospitalist

I have three rules for psychiatry. The staff are sicker than the patients. Don't let the lunatics run the asylum. And don't work harder than the patients work for themselves.
—Bruce Heimer, M.D.
Psychiatrist

She's just old.
—Michael Coleman, D.O.
Family physician

Chapter 1

A Young Tragedy

I can still remember Ms. Osborne's long, messy, brown hair and pale, attractive face like it was yesterday. She was young, and she presented to the Brighton Medical Center Emergency Department (ED) unconscious after an OxyContin overdose. I saw her as soon as she arrived with Brent Johnson, a young, trim, handsome M.D. who was wearing hunter green scrubs embroidered with his name, degree, and "Emergency Medicine" on the left of the shirt.

Two paramedics rushed Ms. Osborne into the ED on a gurney, and a disheveled, panicked, older woman was with them. The female paramedic was holding a bag valve mask over Ms. Osborne's nose and mouth. The bag had a line connected to an oxygen tank, and the paramedic rhythmically squeezed the bag to ventilate the patient.

"Ms. Osborne is 23 years old," the male paramedic said. "Her mother found her down in her room with a half-empty bottle of OxyContin, a syringe, and needle beside her. She doesn't know how long she was down, and she was unable to arouse her. When we arrived, she was cyanotic with agonal breathing, pinpoint pupils, and her pulse ox was 35.[1] She didn't respond to two milligrams of Narcan.[2] Pulse ox is now 93, BP 102 over 68. Pulse is 129."

The paramedics moved her limp body from the gurney to a bed in a private room. I grabbed the bag valve mask to continue ventilation. A nurse quickly connected Ms. Osborne to hospital oxygen and a vitals monitor. The monitor alarm dinged due to tachycardia (rapid heart rate). The paramedics told the woman they were sorry, and they left. Ms. Osborne gasped and snorted at times between breaths I gave her.

1

Dr. Johnson opened her eyelids. Her pupils were dilated, and they didn't respond to a penlight. He palpated her radial pulse in a wrist.

"Let's give her another two milligrams of Narcan IM,"[3] he said. The nurse was prepared with a syringe of the medication, and she gave her the injection in the deltoid muscle of a shoulder.

"You're her mother?" Dr. Johnson said.

"Yes," the woman said with tears in her eyes.

"Okay. I'm Dr. Johnson. Do you know how long she was in her room?"

"Maybe an hour or two. I don't know for sure. She spends a lot of time in her room. She just moved back in with me to try to get back on her feet, and she said she was going to stay clean this time. I made dinner, and she didn't answer when I called her for dinner. So I went to check on her, and she was passed out. Her skin was blue, and she wasn't breathing at first, but then she started gasping. I shook her and slapped her, but I couldn't wake her up."

"Do you know if she used anything else besides OxyContin?"

"I don't think so, but I don't know for sure."

"Do you know if she's used other drugs before like Xanax, Ativan, Klonopin, or Valium?"[4]

"She's used Xanax and who knows what else. Is she going to be okay!"

"She's not responding to another dose of Narcan."

She started to cry. "Please help her! She's my baby, and she's got three kids!"

"I'm really sorry. This is terrible." He pressed one of her fingernails with his fingernail, then made a fist and rubbed her sternum with his knuckles. "She's also not responding to pain."

She cried harder. "Please help her! She's my baby!"

"Let's give her another dose of Narcan IV. She needs a blood drug screen, CMP, and CBC."[5]

The nurse rushed to get the medication and supplies for the IV and labs.

The mother stroked her daughter's hair with tears streaming down her face. "I love you, Christine. Please wake up. Your children need you."

The nurse had difficulty placing the IV. She stuck her several times in the antecubital area of her right forearm (anterior to the elbow), but she couldn't access a vein, and she couldn't find a suitable vein to try in the other forearm. She found a vein in the right dorsal hand, and she was able to establish the line after a couple of sticks. She drew three vials of blood for labs and administered IV Narcan.

Christine's condition remained unchanged after a few minutes. She continued to gasp and snort at times between the breaths that I gave her, and the monitor alarm continued to ding.

"You have to wake up, Christine," her mother said. "Your children need you, and I love you so much."

Dr. Johnson ordered more doses of Narcan, but Christine still didn't respond. He checked her pain response and her pupils with a penlight again.

"Come on, Christine!" her mother said. "Wake up! You can't do this!" She shook her by a shoulder.

"Her drug screen was positive for OxyContin and Klonopin," Dr. Johnson said. "Klonopin is long-acting, so she could have taken a dose a few days ago, and the medication would still be in her system. The combination of OxyContin and Klonopin is very dangerous, especially with IV use. The drugs may have stopped her breathing long enough to cause brain damage."

"What does that mean!"

"She's probably not responding to Narcan because her brain has been damaged from prolonged lack of oxygen. She's still not breathing on her own, which means that the respiratory center in her brainstem may be damaged."

"But she's taking some breaths."

"She's not taking real breaths. She has agonal respiration, which is caused by a brainstem reflex."

"Well, can't you put her on a breathing machine?"

"Yes. We can intubate her, put her on ventilator, and admit her to the ICU, but she may not be able to come off the ventilator."

"So she'd be a vegetable!"

"She may not come out of a coma."

"Well, I want her put on a breathing machine."

"Okay." Dr. Johnson intubated her (placed a breathing tube in her trachea), connected her to a ventilator, and adjusted the settings.

She wailed. "You can't do this, Christine! You hear me! You have to wake up!" She shook her by a shoulder again. "You have to wake up! Wake up!" She stroked her hair and kissed her cheek. "I should have found you sooner. I'm sorry. I love you so much."

Dr. Johnson and I went back to the "doc box," a long, narrow room behind the nurses' station in the center of the ED. The room had a long, built-in desk with computers, and two other doctors were in the room. Dr. Johnson sat in front of his computer. His shoulders slumped, and he sighed. I sat next to him.

"Fuck," Dr. Johnson said. "Another casualty of hillbilly heroin. Her poor kids."

"I'm sorry," I said. "This is a terrible case."

"Yeah. At least she won't die in the ED."

"You think she's going to die?"

"Yes."

"Did you consider using flumazenil?"[6]

"Flumazenil is contraindicated with mixed overdoses, and it can cause seizures and ventricular arrhythmias."[7]

"Okay."

Christine Osborne was quickly admitted to the ICU.

Endnotes

1. Cyanotic: bluish skin from lack of oxygen. Agonal breathing: abnormal, inadequate pattern of gasping, labored breathing. A pulse oximeter measures oxygen saturation in arterial blood noninvasively, using a device on a finger or ear lobe. Normal readings are 95–100%.

2. Narcan (naloxone) is the antidote for opioid overdose.

3. IM: intramuscular.

4. Xanax, Ativan, Klonopin, and Valium are benzodiazepines, a class of controlled, addictive medications that have antianxiety, hypnotic, antiepileptic, and skeletal muscle relaxant effects. Benzodiazepines increase risk of lethal respiratory depression in combination with opioids.

5. CMP: comprehensive metabolic panel is a lab that measures electrolytes, glucose (blood sugar), kidney, and liver function. CBC: complete blood cell count.

6. Flumazenil is an antidote for benzodiazepine overdoses.

7. Ventricular arrhythmias are types of abnormal heart rhythms.

Chapter 2

Twists and Turns

I attended the Brighton College School of Osteopathic Medicine (BCSOM), and I saw Ms. Osborne during my first emergency medicine rotation at the beginning of my fourth and final, glorious year of medical school. At the time, I had senioritis. I just wanted to match with a good psychiatry residency and graduate. But I had to trudge through more rotations, and I was battling anxiety and pessimism. I had just received a rejection from one of the residency programs I applied to, and I had a bad feeling in the pit of my stomach that I had just failed the $1,100 Comprehensive Osteopathic Medical Licensing Examination (COMLEX) Level 2-Performance Evaluation. The Level 2-PE was a nerve-wracking, seven-hour exam, playing doctor with 12 actor patients in Philadelphia. I had to pass it to graduate, and I had to wait 8–10 weeks for the result! Failure was not an option. I had to become a doctor to repay $230,000 in student loans, and the loans had a 6.875% interest rate ($16,000 per year).

BCSOM was in Brighton, a rural town of 6,636 residents in the Appalachian Mountains of Eastern Kentucky, a region stricken with poverty, a high unemployment rate, and an opioid epidemic. My wife, Lynn, and I lived in a subsidized apartment complex that was riddled with riffraff (alcoholics, addicts, drug dealers, and thieves). The journey through my third and fourth clinical years of medical school was remarkable, full of twists, turns, intellectual and emotional challenges that tested my fortitude. I encountered a motley cast of patients and doctors—including a patient with blue skin and a hostile, tantrum-throwing ob-gyn—who taught me how to become a physician. I saw the best and worst in humanity and even patients who have seen glimpses of heaven and hell.

Chapter 3

Family Medicine

My third year started on the first sweltering Monday of August with a two-month family medicine rotation with Michael Coleman, D.O. I'd survived the first two rigorous years of medical school to get to this point and passed my COMLEX Level 1, my first medical licensing exam. Many people don't know what a doctor of osteopathic medicine (D.O.) is because most physicians are M.D.s, but the osteopathic profession has grown exponentially since 1980 with the addition of many new schools, branch campuses, and increased class sizes. In 1980 D.O.s only constituted 4% of U.S. physicians (17,620). In 2010 they constituted 7% (63,000), and by 2020 they had grown to 13% (120,500). My osteopathic medicine rotation is covered in the next chapter. Osteopathy has a storied history that began with an eccentric "lightning bonesetter" in 1874.

A family medicine doctor has to know a little bit about everything, like a jack-of-all-trades. Dr. Coleman worked in a nice, large clinic in Branham that was owned by Appalachian Valley Medical Center (AVMC), a 164-bed hospital. He and his partner, Sean Hunt, D.O., were graduates of BCSOM's first class in 2000, and they had been practicing for five years since they completed a three-year residency. Branham was half an hour from Brighton, and it was half the size of Brighton with a population of 3,125.

On my way to the clinic, I heard a radio ad with the voice of Eric C. Conn, the "Mr. Social Security" attorney, urging people to call him to "get the disability you deserve." I also passed one of his fluorescent yellow, gaudy billboards, which had a large image of him and said he was "Kentucky's One & Only Board-Certified Social Security Disability Specialist." Eastern

Kentucky's highways were blanketed with his billboards, and radio and TV stations frequently played his ads, extolling Conn as the region's preeminent, bilingual disability expert. I wondered how many able-bodied people were on "the draw" (receiving disability checks).

I arrived at the clinic front desk at 8 a.m., and a nurse took me to Dr. Coleman's large office. His office was furnished with a large, beautiful rosewood desk, a large, matching bookcase filled with medical textbooks and journals, and luxurious, leather chairs. Fox News was on a TV on his wall, showing coverage of the 2008 presidential race (Obama vs. McCain). Dr. Coleman was sitting at his desk, looking at a computer screen. He appeared young, wearing a stethoscope around his neck, a white Oxford shirt, and khaki pants.

"Dr. Coleman. Good morning," I said. "I'm James Banks."

"Hi, James," he said. "Man, you're tall. Have a seat. I'm just checking my schedule. I have a couple of patients waiting. Where are you from?"

"Tennessee. How about you?" I sat in a very comfortable chair in front of his desk.

"Born and raised in Branham. Do you know what you want to go into?"

"Psychiatry, I think. I just need to do a psychiatry rotation to be sure I like the clinical aspect of it."

"We could use a psychiatrist here."

"Really?"

"Yeah. We don't have anyone in Branham to refer to. It's hard to get patients into MBHS in Brighton, and care there is hit or miss."

"What's MBHS?"

"Mountain Behavioral Health Services. You could make more money, working with us."

"How's that?"

"We have a higher Medicaid reimbursement rate, so you'd make more than you would if you hung up your own shingle."

"Okay."

"I'm serious. We could make you an offer."

"Well, I've still got two years of medical school and four years of residency ahead of me."

"So you'll have plenty of time to think about it." He smiled.

I smiled back. It felt good to be discussing a potential job opportunity so soon, but I couldn't imagine myself living in Branham.

He rose from his desk. "We've got all kinds of pathology. You can start reviewing charts while I go see these patients real quick." He left his office.

I sat at his desk and reviewed the chart of a 67-year-old female with chief complaint of dizziness. I wasn't familiar with the electronic medical record (EMR) system, so I had to spend some time figuring out how to find important information, like chief complaint, vital signs, weight, diagnoses, medication list, labs, and other tests. EMRs were designed by information technology professionals for billing, so they weren't user-friendly for doctors. I was still reviewing the chart when Dr. Coleman returned.

"Who's next?" he said.

"Velma Hatfield," I said. "She's a 67-year-old female with dizziness."

"Okay. Go see her, and I'll join you in a few minutes."

"Okay." I rose from his desk.

He looked at the TV, which showed Obama at a campaign rally with a large, enthusiastic crowd. "Lord help us if Obama wins," he said. "He's a commie."

I laughed and left his office to see the patient in a small exam room. She appeared her stated age, petite, well-groomed and well-dressed, sitting in a chair. I sat on a rolling stool in front of her.

"Ms. Hatfield. Hello," I said. "I'm James. I'm a medical student."

"What was that?" she said.

"I'm James," I said louder. "I'm a medical student."

"Hi, James," she said.

"You sound congested."

"Yeah. It's hard to breathe through my nose, and I'm dizzy and not hearing so well."

"When did the dizziness start?"

"About a week ago."

"Have you felt lightheaded, like you might faint?"

"No."

"Have you felt like the room's moving or like you're on a boat?" I was trying to distinguish dizziness from vertigo.

"No. I just feel dizzy."

"Okay. Have you had any falls?"

"Well, I almost fell when I felt real dizzy the other day. I stumbled a little bit, but I caught myself."

"Okay. Your blood pressure looks good. How long have you been congested?"

"Maybe two to three weeks. I've got bad allergies."

"Have you taken anything for it?"

"Sudafed and Claritin, but they haven't helped much."

"How long have you had hearing difficulty?"

"That started about the same time as the dizziness."

"Okay. Could you have a seat on the table?"

"Sure." She sat on the table.

I rose from the stool to examine her. I palpated her neck to check for enlarged lymph nodes. I used the light from an otoscope to examine her throat, then I used the instrument to examine her nasal cavity and eardrums.

Dr. Coleman entered the room. "Velma, how are you?" He shook her hand and touched her shoulder.

"Not so good," she said. "That's why I'm here."

"I'm sorry you don't feel well," he said. "How are the grandkids?"

"They're doing okay, I guess. Now that they're in their twenties, they seem to be too busy for their grandmother."

"That sounds about right." He turned to me. "James, what's going on with her?"

"She's been congested for two to three weeks due to allergies," I said. "Sudafed and Claritin have been ineffective. She's had dizziness and difficulty hearing for one week, and she had a near fall. She's normotensive. Her oropharynx is erythematous[1] without exudate. Nasopharynx is erythematous and edematous.[2] And it looks like she has fluid behind both tympanic membranes."

"Let me take a look." He examined her throat, nasal cavity, and eardrums. "You do have bilateral effusion, so it's no wonder you're dizzy and can't hear well. What should we do with her, James?" He smiled at her.

"How about Flonase and an oral steroid?" I said.

"Sounds like a plan," he said. "We'll get you a Medrol Dosepak." He sat on the stool and turned to the computer on a small desk to order her medications and complete her visit note. He smiled at her again and touched her arm. "I hope you get to feeling better soon." Dr. Coleman and I left the room.

I only saw four other patients on my first day with Dr. Coleman because he had been on call the night before, so he only worked a half day. I saw a 53-year-old male for a hypertension (HTN) reassessment, an 18-year-old female with abdominal pain and ovarian cysts, a 51-year-old male with diarrhea and excess gas, and a 71-year-old obese female with rheumatoid arthritis and left knee pain. She was scheduled for a knee replacement.

Dr. Coleman and Dr. Hunt rounded on their own patients at AVMC, so their days were very busy as they rushed to and from the hospital between seeing lots of patients in their clinic. Established patients in their clinic had 15-minute appointments, and new patients had 30-minute appointments. The doctors often had some double bookings, so they usually saw 30 or more outpatients per day.

When I returned to our apartment, I passed a young man who lived in our building. He appeared disheveled, dirty, and intoxicated as usual. He had approached Lynn and me one day as we were going into our apartment, and he told us he could get us pills if we wanted them.

Tuesday was a reading day because Dr. Coleman attended the memorial service for Dean Brown, who had been BCSOM's associate dean of student affairs. Dean Brown had been morbidly obese (body mass index greater than 40) and ill-appearing. He had a thick beard and tobacco stains around his mouth, and he had enjoyed smoking his pipe in his office. I couldn't believe he was allowed to smoke in his office, which was, of course, saturated with the smell. At least pipe smoke smelled better than cigar or cigarette smoke. Dean Brown died of cardiac arrest at age 59. I was impressed he had lived that long.

For my reading I selected type 2 diabetes mellitus (DM) from *Harrison's Principles of Internal Medicine*, 16th edition. DM was common in Eastern Kentucky because most people were overweight or obese. Management of DM could be challenging — especially when many of the patients were noncompliant with medications and diet and exercise recommendations. Glucose-lowering agents included insulin and four classes of oral hypoglycemics: insulin secretagogues (sulfonylureas and meglitinides), biguanide (metformin), α-glucosidase inhibitors, and insulin sensitizers (thiazolidinediones).

Wednesday was much busier. I saw 14 patients, including two in AVMC. The first outpatient of the day was a 63-year-old female who was stable on immunosuppressive medications (Prograf and CellCept) for a liver transplant she had nine years earlier. She had contracted hepatitis A in 7th grade, and the virus slowly destroyed her liver over the decades.

We also saw a 28-year-old opioid addict for his initial Suboxone[3] appointment. He was sitting in a chair in the exam room. He appeared older than his stated age and underweight with sunken cheeks. He was unshaven, with disheveled, dirty blond hair, wearing a tattered T-shirt and jeans.

"Anthony, good morning. I'm Dr. Coleman, and this is James."

"Nice to meet you," he said.

"Hi," I said.

"How are you?" Dr. Coleman sat on a rolling stool.

"I've been better," Anthony said. "I'm glad I could get in here to see you."

"Okay. You're here for a Suboxone appointment?"

"Yeah."

"Okay. Tell me what you've been using."

"I've been using Subutex[4] to try to get off the other pills."

"Okay. I can't prescribe Subutex for you. Hopefully, they told you that when you made your appointment."

"Yeah. The lady told me that."

"I only prescribe Subutex for pregnant patients with opioid dependence. Are you pregnant?"

"No."

"Okay. Good." Dr. Coleman smiled brightly and slapped Anthony's knee. "When did you last take Subutex?"

"This morning."

"How much?"

"One tab, but I don't think it's enough. My cravings are through the roof."

"Okay. How did you take the medication?"

"Like it's supposed to be taken."

"Have you snorted or injected it before?"

"Yeah, but I stopped doing that."

"Have you injected it?"

"Yeah."

"When did you last inject it?"

"About a month ago."

"Okay. Let me see your arms."

Anthony raised his arms, and Dr. Coleman examined his forearms, which had needle marks.

"What other pills have you been using?" Dr. Coleman said.

"Percs, Roxis, Oxys,"[5] Anthony said.

"Did you inject those too?"

"Yeah."

"Have you been screened for hepatitis and HIV before?"

"No. I need to do that."

"I can order labs for you. Your blood pressure's okay. Do you have any medical conditions like diabetes or high cholesterol?"

"Not that I know of, but I haven't seen a doctor since I was in high school."

"Are you working?"

"I do odd jobs, but I need to find something more steady."

"A full-time job could help to keep you out of trouble. Idle hands are the Devil's workshop. Let me take a listen to you." Dr. Coleman auscultated the patient's heart with his stethoscope, scooted his stool to the computer desk, completed the history and physical note, and ordered Suboxone. "Okay. You can pick up your prescription up front, and you need to follow up with me in one week to get your next prescription."

"Okay. Thank you." Anthony pulled several hundred-dollar bills out of his wallet.

"You don't pay me. You pay up front."

"Okay." Anthony put the cash back in his pocket.

Dr. Coleman stood to leave the room. "You better not bullshit me 'cause if you do, I'll kick you out. You understand?"

"Yeah."

"Okay. Stay out of trouble." Dr. Coleman touched his shoulder, and we returned to his office.

"What do you charge for Suboxone appointments?" I said.

"Two-fifty for the first appointment, then one hundred for follow-ups," Dr. Coleman said.

"Wow. So he'll pay *five hundred fifty dollars* for his first month of treatment if he's following up weekly."

"Yeah, and the medication's not cheap either. But if he does well, I'll stretch out his appointments to every two weeks after two to three months."

"Okay. I wonder how he'll afford that if he's just doing odd jobs."

"That's not my business. All of our Suboxone patients pay cash because insurance won't cover the treatment. Hillbilly heroin is a big problem around here."

"What's hillbilly heroin?"

"OxyContin. There are a lot of pill mills around here. The Kentucky attorney general and eight counties have even filed a class-action lawsuit against Purdue Pharma, seeking millions for drug rehab programs and law enforcement. The jail in Brighton wasn't big enough, so they had to spend $6.5 million to make it bigger. Five current and former Purdue executives have pleaded guilty to misleading the public about OxyContin's risk of addiction."

We saw a few more patients, then rushed to the hospital in Dr. Coleman's Cadillac Escalade. As he sped toward the hospital, my back pressed deeper into the luxurious leather seat when he accelerated quickly, and my torso was pulled from side to side as he took fast turns. I was actually a little anxious but comforted by being in a large vehicle. We would probably be okay if we were in a crash.

"Wow," I said. "You drive fast."

"I'm a busy doctor." He smiled.

"You don't seem to be concerned about getting a speeding ticket."

"The cops know me."

"That must be nice. Does Dr. Hunt drive like this too?"

"Oh, he's worse than me. Don't ride with him."

"Got it."

The hospital cases weren't interesting. We saw a 57-year-old female with abdominal pain and a 56-year-old female who was recovering from surgery for a humerus fracture. Dr. Coleman discharged both patients. We sped back to the clinic, and we had lunch in the break room before seeing more patients. Pharmaceutical representatives provided lunch nearly every day, which was a nice perk for a poor medical student. We had a nice spread of food from a Mexican restaurant: chicken and beef tacos, enchiladas, tamales, and chocolate-dipped churros for dessert. I enjoyed a couple of tasty tamales and a churro. Then I wanted to take a nap, but I pushed through my lethargy to see more patients.

The last patient of the day was a new patient, a 50-year-old male who appeared thin, pale, ill. He had fecal incontinence with blood in his stools for the past month, and he had lost 20 pounds over the past eight months. He hadn't seen a doctor in years, and he didn't like to see doctors. His BP was 98/68. Dr. Coleman advised him to drink plenty of fluids, including some Gatorade, to stay well hydrated, and he referred him for a colonoscopy, which would probably show advanced colon cancer.

The clinic was busy again on Thursday, and no patients were in the hospital. On Friday I only saw three patients because Dr. Coleman worked half days on Fridays, but one of the cases was interesting.

John May was 35 years old, and he appeared older than his stated age, tall, and thin, sitting in a chair in a small exam room. He had Marfan syndrome, a rare, connective tissue multisystemic disorder characterized by musculoskeletal, ocular (lens dislocation, retinal detachment), and cardiovascular abnormalities. The syndrome is an autosomal dominant inherited disorder, and approximately 20% of cases are caused by new mutations. John had required surgeries for aortic valve replacement and aortic dissection, which extended from the arch of the aorta to the iliac artery (top to bottom of aorta). It was amazing he was still alive!

"John. Hello," I said. "I'm James. I'm a medical student."

"Hi, James," he said. "I think I've met about all of the students who have been here."

"Because you have Marfan syndrome?" I sat on a rolling stool in front of him.

"Yeah. I'm a special case."

"Do you get tired of all the students seeing you?"

"I don't mind."

"Okay. Did either of your parents have Marfan syndrome?"

"My mom did. She died when I was 16."

"I'm sorry."

"Thanks."

"How did she die?"

"Her aorta ruptured."

"Well, considering you had an aortic dissection, you're lucky to still be alive."

"I'm blessed."

"Yes. How are you doing?"

"Okay."

"You're here for a routine follow-up?"

"Yeah."

"You take Coreg?"[6]

"Yes."

"Your blood pressure and pulse are low. Have you had any dizziness or lightheadedness?"

"Sometimes I get a little lightheaded if I get up too quick."

"Have you had any falls?"

"No."

"Okay. Could you take your shirt off?"

"Sure." He removed his shirt.

I observed pectus excavatum (sunken chest). I palpated his radial pulse and auscultated his heart and lungs. "You can put your shirt back on."

"Okay." He put his shirt back on.

Dr. Coleman entered the room. "Hey, John. What's going on?"

"Not much," John said.

"How's your wife?"

"Good."

"Good. Have you been taking your Coreg?"

"Yes."

"Not missing any doses?"

"No."

"Good. And you haven't been doing anything strenuous?"

"No. I take it easy."

"Good." Dr. Coleman turned to me. "I've commended John for wanting to work, but I've told him he can't work. He's on disability."

"His blood pressure's 96 over 68, and his pulse is 65," I said. "He sometimes gets lightheaded when he rises too quickly, but he hasn't had any falls."

"That's okay. We want to keep his blood pressure and heart rate low so he doesn't have another aortic dissection. Good to see you, John. Tell your wife I said hi."

"I will," John said.

Dr. Coleman and I left the room. I returned home early and took a nap on the couch.

Lynn returned to our apartment shortly after 5 p.m., and she disturbed my nap. Lynn worked as a teller for First Kentucky Bank.

"Hey, babe," I said.

"Hey," she said, "How long have you been home?"

"A few hours. Dr. Coleman works half days on Fridays."

"That must be nice."

"Yeah. Dr. Coleman's cool, and drug reps provide lunch every day."

"Well, I had to deal with some real assholes today. I'm so glad it's the weekend."

"Sorry, babe."

"Yeah. I am so over this job." Lynn frequently complained about work.

"I know. Well, we can have a nice, relaxing weekend."

"I need a beer."

During my second week Dr. Coleman allowed me to perform osteopathic manipulative treatment (OMT) on a 33-year-old female who had low back pain with radiation to her left toes. She injured her back four years earlier when she lifted an 80-pound box of hamburger meat in a nursing home. I was glad I was able to ease her pain.

We also saw a 71-year-old male with a mass on his left adrenal gland (which sits on top of the kidney). He had been having intermittent episodes with headaches, palpitations, sweating, and severe hypertension, so labs were ordered—a plasma metanephrine level and 24-hour urine for catecholamines, vanillylmandelic acid,[7] and metanephrine. The plasma metanephrine level was normal, but the 24-hour urine levels were elevated, so an abdominal CT scan was ordered, and the imaging showed the mass.

"What's the diagnosis?" Dr. Coleman asked me.

"Pheochromocytoma," I said. I remembered the rare catecholamine-secreting tumor because I had joked with my classmate Chris Devlin about how it was his favorite disease ever since he learned about it in pathology.

"Good. What's the treatment?"

"Surgery."

"Yes."

I saw more hospital cases with Dr. Coleman on Wednesday. One of the patients was a 93-year-old female with dyspnea (shortness of breath) and chest pain. I was thinking critically about likely causes of her symptoms like a good medical student.

"She's just old," Dr. Coleman said.

I laughed. "She is pretty old."

On Thursday in the clinic, I saw a 66-year-old female with ulcerative colitis, a permanent colostomy,[8] a gastric ulcer, and hiatal hernia. I was impressed with how well she coped with having a colostomy bag to collect her feces for the rest of her life. I saw a 56-year-old female with severe COPD,[9] dyspnea, and pitting leg edema (pressing tissue with a finger left a temporary depression, a sign of right heart failure). She had a respiratory rate of 24 (normal is 12–20) and a pulse ox of 90% (normal is above 95%) on four liters of oxygen by nasal cannula. I couldn't believe she wasn't in an ED. I also couldn't believe she continued to smoke cigarettes! Near the end of the day, I saw a 19-year-old male with auditory hallucinations who had been sexually abused by an uncle. He continued to intermittently use marijuana, even though Dr. Coleman repeatedly advised him to stop using the substance because it worsened hallucinations and caused paranoia and panic attacks.

On Friday Dr. Coleman told me I didn't have to come in for a half day, so I read about thyroid disorders.

During my third week I started following hospital cases. Dr. Coleman gave me his password so I could log in to hospital computers to review patient charts. He sent me to AVMC ahead of him, and I was anxious about seeing inpatients on my own for the first time. I drove to the hospital at a reasonable speed since I didn't know the cops, and I sat in front of a computer at a nurses' station on the second floor to review charts. I was thankful that the nurses were very friendly and helpful. I had to spend some time familiarizing myself with the EMR. My patient list included a 41-year-old female with breast cancer, nausea, vomiting, pain; a 61-year-old female with type 1 DM, dialysis, vomiting, fever; a 78-year-old female unable to ambulate (walk); and a 91-year-old female with chest pain.

The patient with breast cancer was reclined in bed with the head tilted up, watching a morning show on TV. She appeared her stated age, thin, wearing a colorful headscarf and hospital gown, and she had an IV line connected to a bag of normal saline.

"Ms. McCoy. Hello," I said. "I'm James. I'm a medical student."

"Hi, James," she said. "Who are you with? I have so many doctors, it's hard to keep up with them all."

"Dr. Coleman."

"Oh, he's wonderful."

"He is a good doctor. So you've had a mastectomy for breast cancer, and now you're having chemo?"

"Yes. And it's made me so sick, I wished I was dead."

"I'm sorry."

"Me too."

"You've been having nausea, vomiting, and pain?"

"Yes."

"Where is the pain?"

"Well, of course, I've had some pain from the surgery, but then I had pain all over, and I couldn't even keep water down before I was put back in the hospital."

"Your labs indicate you were dehydrated when you were readmitted, and you've received IV fluids. How are you feeling now?"

"Much better. I still have some pain, but it's a lot better, and I haven't thrown up again."

"So the Percocet and Zofran[10] have helped?"

"Yes. Now if I could just get something for my chemo brain."

"What do you mean?"

"I've been forgetting things, and I can't concentrate. It's a lot harder to get things done now."

"Sorry. I don't think we can help you with that."

"I figured I'll just have to deal with it. I'd like to go home today."

"Well, your labs look better. Have you been able to eat and drink?"

"Yes."

"Good. Well, I'll let Dr. Coleman know you're ready to go home. Is it okay if I examine you?"

"Sure."

I palpated her radial pulse, auscultated her heart and lungs, and pressed on her abdomen. "Dr. Coleman will see you soon."

"Okay. Thank you."

"You're welcome."

The patient reminded me of my mother, who died of metastatic breast cancer at age 43. I saw her shortly before she died in the hospital, where she was receiving radiation treatment. It was very difficult to see a wonderful, intelligent woman withered away to skin and bones. She was delirious with slurred speech, and she had grand-mal seizures. She had been the only professor at the small Christian university who taught math, physics, and computer science. She was working on her Ph.D., and she taught Bible classes. While she was lucid, I told her I planned to become a doctor.

My father held her left hand during her last moments, fulfilling a promise he had made to her. He asked her if she could see Jesus coming for her, and she said, "It could be. I see silvery waves." These were her last words before she lost consciousness and faded away. Her hand grew cold, and my father continued to hold it until about half an hour after her heart stopped.

My mother was a quiet woman, but about 1,000 people attended her funeral at our church, which was a testament to how loving and selfless she was. I loved my mother very much, and I missed her. She was an angel on Earth, and I liked to think that she could see me in medical school from Heaven.

I left the patient's room and went to see the 61-year-old female with type 1 DM, dialysis, vomiting, and fever. She was sitting up in bed, watching TV. She appeared older than her stated age, pale, ill, wearing a hospital gown, and she had an IV line. She was on long-term dialysis because years of poorly controlled glucose destroyed her kidneys. I thought about how miserable life would be chained to a dialysis machine three days a week. Noncompliance with dialysis treatment would lead to death in one to three weeks.

I was intimidated by diabetes management—especially for a type 1 diabetic with dialysis and fever. She could have bacteremia (bacteria in the blood) from the dialysis. Blood cultures were pending, and she had been given vancomycin and ceftazidime, broad-spectrum antibiotics for empiric coverage of gram-positive and gram-negative bacteria. She was on scheduled long-acting and regular insulin, and sliding-scale insulin could be used if her glucose wasn't adequately controlled. She had other abnormal lab values, but I didn't know what was considered normal for a patient on dialysis. I knew anemia was common with chronic kidney disease, and blood urea nitrogen (BUN) and creatinine levels increased between dialysis treatments.

"Ms. Justice. Hello," I said. "I'm James. I'm a medical student working with Dr. Coleman."

"Hi, James," she said.

"How are you?"

"I've been better."

"You have type 1 diabetes, you're on dialysis, and you were admitted for vomiting and fever?"

"Yes."

"You've received some antibiotics and Zofran, and you haven't had a fever since yesterday afternoon. Have you been able to eat and drink?"

"A little bit. I haven't had much of an appetite."

"Okay. Could I take a look at your fistula?"

"Sure."

I examined her left forearm, and I didn't see any erythema over her arteriovenous fistula,[11] which was used for dialysis. I palpated the thrill (vibration) of the fistula. I auscultated her heart and lungs and pressed on her abdomen. "Dr. Coleman will see you soon."

"Okay. Thank you."

"You're welcome."

I left the room and went to see the 78-year-old female who was unable to ambulate. She was asleep in bed, and she appeared her stated age, obese, pale, wearing a hospital gown. Her right eye was bruised. Her labs were normal, including serial troponins.[12] BP was 103/68, pulse was 66. The computer reading of her EKG showed sinus rhythm and septal myocardial infarction of indeterminate age (heart attack, death of a specific area of heart muscle, usually due to blockage of a coronary artery by a plaque or clot), and I didn't know how to interpret that. Head CT showed mild cerebral atrophy (loss of brain tissue) and no acute intracranial abnormality, but I wondered if she could have a neurological problem that couldn't be detected with a CT.

"Ms. Thacker. Hello," I said.

She didn't move.

"Ms. Thacker," I said louder.

She didn't respond, so I gently touched her shoulder, and she turned toward me.

"Ms. Thacker. Hello. I'm James. I'm a medical student working with Dr. Coleman."

"Hello, James," she said. "I just think the world of Dr. Coleman. Is he teaching you lots?"

"Yes. He is a good doctor. What happened to your eye?"

"I had a fall."

"How did that happen?"

"Well, I was just going to the kitchen to make dinner, and the next thing I knew, I was on the floor. I must have hit my head on the fridge."

"Did you feel dizzy or lightheaded before you fell?"

"No. It just happened. There have been times I've felt dizzy, but I didn't fall."

"Have you had a heart attack in the past or been diagnosed with a heart condition?"

"No."

"Did you have difficulty walking before you fell?"

"No."

"Do you feel like you have a problem with balance or moving your legs?"

"My legs just give out, and I feel weak."

"Okay. Could you try to stand up for me?"

"I can try." She sat up, grabbed the walker, which I placed in front of her, and she slowly stood up beside the bed.

"Do you think you could take a few steps to the door?"

"I don't know. I just feel so weak, like my knees are going to give out." She took a few small, shuffling steps.

"Okay. That's obviously very difficult for you. You can sit back down."

She slowly shuffled backwards and sat down, appearing exhausted.

I palpated her radial pulse, auscultated her heart and lungs, and pressed on her abdomen. "Dr. Coleman will see you soon."

"Thank you."

"You're welcome."

I left the room and went to see Ms. Blackburn, the 91-year-old female with chest pain. She was also asleep, and she appeared heavily wrinkled and frail. Her EKG and serial troponins didn't indicate that she had an MI (myocardial infarction). She had received nitroglycerin, aspirin, Plavix (antiplatelet medication), metoprolol, and morphine. I awakened her to ask how she was feeling, and I examined her, but she was just old.

I went to meet Dr. Coleman at a nurses' station. He was hurriedly reviewing charts on a computer.

"How are our patients doing?" he said.

"Ms. McCoy has breast cancer," I said. "She was admitted for chemotherapy-induced vomiting, dehydration, and pain. She's received IV fluids, Zofran, and Percocet. BUN and creatinine are normal. She's been able to eat and drink, and she's ready to go home.

"Ms. Justice has type 1 diabetes. She's on dialysis for end-stage renal disease, and she was admitted for vomiting and fever. She's received vancomycin, ceftazidime, Zofran. Blood cultures are pending, and she's been afebrile for 16 hours. I palpated her fistula, which was a first for me."

"What did it feel like?" he said.

"Kind of like a purring cat," I said.

"That's a good description."

"Ms. Thacker was admitted for inability to ambulate. Prior to admission she had a fall from a syncopal episode, and she bruised her right eye. She denied feeling dizzy or lightheaded before the fall, and she denied difficulty walking before the fall. She said her legs just give out, and she feels weak. She was only able to take a few small, shuffling steps with a walker, and she was exhausted. Labs are normal, vitals are stable, but her blood pressure and pulse are a bit low. EKG shows sinus rhythm and an old septal infarct, according to the computer reading, but I don't know how to interpret that. She denied history of MI."

"Computer readings are usually crap, but most septal infarcts are silent. Cardiologists and other specialists here don't like me and Dr. Hunt because we don't consult them enough. We can read our own EKGs and manage most of our patients appropriately without specialists. We order consults if we really need them, but unnecessary consults just keep patients in the hospital longer, and the hospital is a dangerous place to be."

"What do you mean by dangerous?"

"Patients get hospital-acquired infections, like pneumonia. Nurses make medication errors. Patients have falls."

"Okay. Ms. Thacker's head CT showed mild cerebral atrophy but nothing acute."

"How old is she?"

"Seventy-eight."

"So the CT is normal for her age. Our brains are shrinking right now as we speak."

"Well, that sucks."

"It does, doesn't it? If I get dementia, I'd rather someone shoot me than put me in a nursing home. Or they could give me too much OxyContin. That would be the best way to go."

"I wouldn't want to be in a nursing home either. But if you're demented, maybe you wouldn't know you're in a nursing home."

"Oh, I would know."

I smiled. "Could Ms. Thacker have a neurological problem that wouldn't show up on the CT?"

"Sure. And an MRI might pick up something missed by the CT, but she may have a problem with her ticker. Maybe she had cardiogenic syncope. If her EKG and telemetry are okay, she may need to wear a Holter monitor."[13]

"Okay. The last patient is Ms. Blackburn, the 91-year-old female with chest pain. She's just old."

Dr. Coleman laughed, and we went to see the patients together. He discharged Ms. McCoy and decided to keep the other patients in the hospital. Ms. Justice needed to be afebrile for 24 hours before discharge. Physical therapy was ordered for Ms. Thacker. No new orders were entered for Ms. Blackburn.

The next day I saw a couple of patients in the clinic, then went to AVMC. Ms. Justice remained afebrile for 39 hours, so she was discharged. Ms. Thacker remained unable to ambulate after a physical therapy session, and telemetry showed no events—BP and pulse remained low normal, and she had no arrhythmia.

"What are we going to do with Ms. Blackburn?" Dr. Coleman said.

"I don't know," I said.

"Neither do I." He laughed. "You're supposed to help me here."

"Well, she hasn't had an MI, but she has unstable angina.[14] I don't know if a cardiologist would cath a 91-year-old."

"Exactly."

We rushed out of the hospital. Dr. Coleman peeled out of the parking lot in his Cadillac Escalade, and I pulled out of the parking like a normal person in my Volvo sedan. I saw a patient in the clinic, then Dr. Coleman grabbed me in the hall, and we went to his office.

"You should see this next one with me," he said. "She's a 66-year-old new patient with chief complaint of low back pain. Look at her KASPER report." He handed me a few pages.

"What's KASPER?" I said.

"It's Kentucky's controlled substance monitoring database."

"Okay."

"This report doesn't look good. She's gotten Percocet, Lortab, and tramadol[15] from five different doctors in Eastern Kentucky over the past few months."

"Whoa."

"Yeah. She's doctor shopping. The nurse entered her medication list, but it doesn't include an opioid. I hate seeing drug seekers. Some of them really suck the energy out of me. Let's go get this over with."

I handed the pages back to Dr. Coleman, and he folded them and put them in his pocket. We entered the exam room. The drug seeker was sitting in a chair, and she appeared her stated age, well-groomed and well-dressed.

"Ms. Stone. Hello. I'm Dr. Coleman, and this is James."

"Nice to meet you," she said.

"How are you?" Dr. Coleman sat on a rolling stool.

"I'm good, thanks. How are you?"

"I'm okay. But if you're good, why are you seeing me?"

She smiled. "Well, I'm not actually good. I guess that's the polite answer. My back's been killing me."

"Okay. What's been going on with your back?"

"Well, it's bothered me for years, but lately the pain has been excruciating and shooting down my legs, and I've had trouble getting around."

"The pain has gone down both legs?"

"Yes, and it's terrible. It's debilitating."

"When your pain's excruciating, how would you rate it on a scale of 1–10 with 10 being most intense?"

"Eleven."

"That must be miserable."

"It is. When it's that bad, I can't get out of bed."

"Did you injure your back?"

"No. I guess I'm just getting old."

"Have you had an x-ray or MRI?"

"Yes. My MRI showed degenerative disc disease."

"Okay. Have you taken anything for pain?"

"I tried over-the-counter stuff, but it didn't do anything, so my doctor had me try Celebrex, but it didn't help either."

"Why are you seeing me instead of your other doctor?"

"I don't care for her, so I wanted to find a better doctor. She only spends five minutes with me, and she doesn't really listen to me. I've heard good things about you." She smiled charismatically.

Dr. Coleman smiled. "Okay. Have you tried anything stronger than Celebrex?"

"I got Percocet from my pain management doctor, and it really gave me some relief. But I had to keep getting injections to get the medication, and the injections didn't help."

"Have you tried physical therapy?"

"Yes, but it just made my back worse."

"Okay. Have you tried a muscle relaxer?"

"I tried Flexeril, but it just knocked me out."

"What about Cymbalta?"

"My doctor wanted me to try that one, but I told her I wasn't depressed. I've never had a problem with depression."

"Cymbalta is used for depression, but it's also FDA-approved for chronic pain, fibromyalgia, and neuropathic pain."

"Well, I don't need an antidepressant. I'm actually afraid of those kinds of medicines. I don't want to go crazy or be a zombie. I just need something stronger for my back."

"Okay. Have you tried Neurontin or Lyrica?"[16]

"I tried Neurontin, but Lyrica was way too expensive. Neurontin made me feel drunk, and my feet swelled up."

"Well, it sounds like you've tried about everything except narcotics."

"Yes. It's been so frustrating. I just need a medicine that's going to work."

"Okay. As for your other medical conditions, you have hypertension, hypothyroidism, and you're taking lisinopril, Synthroid, calcium, and vitamin D?"

"Yes."

"Your blood pressure is good. Are you on any other medications?"

"No. That's it."

"Okay. Stand up for me." Dr. Coleman stood to examine her. She stood slowly, wincing with a hand on her lower back.

"The pain is in your low back?"

"Yes."

Dr. Coleman palpated her low back.

She winced. "Ow. That's really tender."

"Bend over as far as you can to try to touch your toes."

"I'll try." She bent a little, winced, and put a hand on her lower back. "That's as far as I can go."

"Okay. Let's step into the hall and let me see how you walk."

She walked slowly with a limp and returned to the exam room.

"Have a seat on the table."

She sat on the table, and Dr. Coleman completed the physical exam.

"Okay," Dr. Coleman said. "Have you tried nabumetone before?"

"No," she said. "What kind of medicine is that?"

"It's a nonsteroidal anti-inflammatory drug."

"Oh. It's an NSAID?"

"Yes, but it's stronger than other NSAIDs you tried."

"NSAIDs didn't help me at all, so I really don't want to try another one. I need something stronger."

"Okay. I have samples of Lyrica for you to try, and we can see if we can get prior authorization from your insurance for the medication so it will be affordable. And you can try Zanaflex for muscle spasms."

"Isn't Lyrica like Neurontin?"

"It is similar."

"Well, I don't want to try that either after my experience with Neurontin, and I don't want another muscle relaxer that's going to knock me out."

"Zanaflex isn't sedating like Flexeril."

"Can't I just get a little Percocet?"

"I'm sorry. I can't prescribe that for you."

"How about Lortab?"

"Sorry. I can't prescribe that either."

"Why not?"

"I refer patients with chronic pain to pain management. I can refer you to a different pain management doctor."

"But pain management didn't help me before. I just need something that's going to work."

"I'm sorry. I can't prescribe an opioid for you."

"Why can't you help me? My pain is *debilitating*. I just want to be able to function and have a decent quality of life. It's not like I'm some druggie. I know we have a big drug problem around here, but some people really need pain medication."

"I'm sorry."

"A friend of mine gets Lortab from you."

"That may be, but I provide individualized treatment, and I can't prescribe the medication for you."

"I just don't understand. It's not like I'm some druggie. Can you please explain to me why you can't help me?"

"Do you need refills for your medications?"

"Why can't you prescribe a medication that works for a patient with debilitating pain?"

"I'm sorry. I'm not going to argue with you about this."

"I'm not arguing. I just want you to explain to me—"

"Do you need refills for your medications?"

"No. I don't need refills. But I think I deserve an explanation."

"I'm not going to prescribe an opioid for you because your controlled medication report shows that you've received Percocet, Lortab, and tramadol from five different doctors over the past few months."

"What! That can't be right!"

Dr. Coleman pulled the KASPER report out of his pocket. "Your name is Jane Stone. Date of birth June 24, 1942?"

"Yes."

"Was Dr. Munish Trivedi your pain management doctor?"

"Yes."

"This report shows that you received Percocet and Lortab from Dr. Trivedi, you received opioids from four other doctors, and you last received Percocet 17 days ago."

"I told you I received those medications from Dr. Trivedi, but the rest of that information can't be correct. That database must have me mixed up with someone else. I have to get this straightened out."

"The report also shows that refills have been received from three different pharmacies. I can call the pharmacies to see if they got you mixed up with someone else. The last refill was received from Taylor's Pharmacy on Main Street in Brighton."

"I'm not some *druggie*. I just need some *real help*, but I'm obviously not going to get that from you." She stepped off the table.

"Doctor shopping is a felony."

"So you're going to call the law on me?"

"No. But you could end up in jail if you don't stop this."

"I'm just trying to get relief from my pain. If that's a crime, then lock me up." She opened the door and left the exam room.

Dr. Coleman and I left right behind her. We observed her walk down the hall for a moment, and we returned to his office.

"How do you think she was walking when she left, compared to before?" Dr. Coleman said.

"She left in a hurry, and she wasn't limping," I said.

"Exactly. She's healed!" He smiled.

Ms. Stone asked a front desk receptionist if she could talk to Dr. Coleman again, and he declined.

The next patient wasn't dramatic. I saw a 77-year-old female for an INR lab check. She was on Coumadin (anticoagulant also used as rat poison) to reduce the risk of atrial fibrillation (type of arrhythmia) sending a blood clot to her brain and causing a stroke. Her INR was 3.5 (therapeutic range 2.0–3.0). An INR less than 2.0 increases risk of clot formation, and an INR greater than 3.0 increases bleeding risk. I asked her if her diet included any green vegetables like kale, spinach, collard greens, brussels sprouts, broccoli, or asparagus. These vegetables are rich in vitamin K, which can decrease the effectiveness of Coumadin.

Dr. Hunt opened the door to the exam room. He appeared young, handsome, wearing a stethoscope around his neck, royal blue scrubs, and white lab coat. His face was a bit mischievous, which was a contrast to Dr. Coleman's honest face. He had the look of a guy who may have gotten into trouble in school and had lots of girlfriends before he was married. According to Dr. Coleman, Dr. Hunt had marital problems. He had been separated from his wife before, and he liked to have cute female medical students with him. Dr. Coleman was happily married with two kids. Both doctors liked to gossip.

"Hi. Sorry to interrupt," Dr. Hunt said. "James, I've got a case for you to see."

"Okay," I said. I turned to the patient. "Dr. Coleman will be with you shortly."

We left the room and walked down a hall.

"What's going on?" I said before we entered the exam room.

"I heard you're gonna be a shrink," he said.

"That's the plan as long as I like my psych rotation."

"Okay. I just want you to observe."

"Okay."

We entered the exam room, and a bad odor immediately stung my nostrils. The patient was sitting in a chair next to the computer desk. She appeared to be in her 30s or 40s, and she was morbidly obese, disheveled, with long, oily hair, wearing a tattered, dirty, long dress.

"Ms. Belcher, this is James. He's a medical student." Dr. Hunt sat on a rolling stool in front of the computer, next to the patient.

"Hi, James," she said.

"Nice to meet you." I sat in a chair on the opposite wall, facing the patient.

"Have you been taking your medications?" Dr. Hunt said.

"I try to remember to take them," she said.

"You're supposed to be taking lisinopril, metformin, and simvastatin,"[17] he said.

"I don't know the names of the pills. I just know what they look like."

I saw a large bug scurry across a lower part of the opposite wall. It looked like a beetle.

"How often do you forget to take your pills?" Dr. Hunt said.

"Oh, I don't know," she said. "Some days I remember. Some days I don't."

"Well, your blood pressure's high, and your A1c[18] and cholesterol are high. You have to take your medications every day for them to work for your blood pressure, diabetes, and cholesterol."

"I know. I'll try to do better."

I saw another bug scurry across the floor. It looked like a roach. Were the bugs coming from the patient! If so, was she unaware or unconcerned that the insects were on her!

"Okay. I'll see you back in 3 months," Dr. Hunt said.

The patient left the room.

"I saw a couple of bugs," I said. "Were they coming from the patient!"

"Well, I didn't see any bugs in the room before she was here," he said.

"Wow!"

"She lives in a shack on the side of a mountain with no electricity or running water."

"I didn't know people still lived like that."

"Yeah. She *really* needs to see a psychiatrist. We need some Lysol in here."

We left the room, and I went to see a 45-year-old male who had been started on Lasix (diuretic) for ankle edema. He had Wernicke aphasia (language impairment), following a stroke that also left him with right-sided hemiplegia (paralysis). He was in a wheelchair, and he appeared his stated age, well-groomed, casually dressed. Wernicke aphasia (also called fluent aphasia or sensory aphasia) is caused by damage to the Wernicke area of the brain, which encompasses a large region of the cerebral cortex of the parietal and temporal lobes. A patient affected with the condition can't comprehend spoken and written words, so speech is fluent but nonsensical.

"Mr. Adkins. Hello," I said. "I'm James. I'm a medical student." I sat on a rolling stool, facing him.

"I'm okay," he said. "I take the car for room with clouds weather you see."

"I'm sorry. Could you say that again?"

"Clouds weather for it over there, over there you see."

"You're saying it's cloudy outside?"

He appeared frustrated. "No. I need my correspondence drawers."

"Your correspondence drawers?"

"Yes. My correspondence drawers." He removed his glasses with his left hand to show me what he was referring to, and he looked at me like I was an idiot. "I can't see without them." He put his glasses back on.

"Okay. How have your ankles been since you started Lasix?"

He appeared irritated. "Why don't you tell me monopoly? They don't show a damn thing. They're making it out for a ride right now, and this is a ride worth waiting for. Shannon calls me from time to time. I'm out with them. Other people are waiting with them and them, and I like being with them. And this one woman, man, she is *really fine* and satisfied. And I like to fish. They're in the weeds, and I use my hands. I save a lot of hands on hold for peoples for us or their hands. I don't know what you get, but I talk with a lot of ham for ham. Sometime and I talk of any more to say am."

"Okay. Your blood pressure looks good. I'd like to take a look at your ankles."

He relaxed. "We'll finally make it."

I examined his ankles. "Dr. Coleman will be in shortly."

"Thank you very much. I appreciate it, and I hope the world lasts for you."

I left the room. I thought about how I would probably rather be dead than have Wernicke aphasia.

The next day was busy. I saw four patients in the clinic in the morning, then went to see seven hospital cases. Ms. Thacker was still unable to ambulate after another physical therapy session. Ms. Blackburn had episodic chest pain at rest that was relieved by nitroglycerin and morphine, and she was able to ambulate slowly with a walker. Dr. Coleman decided to keep her in the hospital for another day. I returned to the clinic to see a few more patients.

The last patient was an 86-year-old female who looked like death. She appeared thin, frail, cyanotic (bluish skin from lack of oxygen), wearing oxygen by nasal cannula. She had congestive heart failure (CHF), COPD, type 2 DM, HTN, hyperlipidemia (HLD), left eye blindness, glaucoma, gout, and rosacea (inflammatory skin disorder). Her cheeks were red with dilated vessels from the rosacea, contrasting with her bluish skin. I thought the poor woman was cursed, and her suffering would be over soon. I felt strong empathy for her, and I was impressed with her perseverance.

"Oh, honey," she said. "I just hand it all over to the Lord, and he helps me along. I'm at peace, and I'm not afraid of dying. The Lord will take me when he's ready, and I'm looking forward to meeting Jesus."

The following morning in the clinic, I saw a 57-year-old male with acromegaly (rare hormonal disorder), weakness, and diarrhea. The skin of his face was coarse, his brows and lower jaw protruded, his nose and lips were large, and he had big hands and feet. Ninety-nine percent of acromegaly cases are caused by growth hormone (GH)-secreting pituitary tumors in the brain. Rarely, acromegaly is caused by a GH-secreting tumor in another location. This patient had transsphenoidal surgery through his nose to remove the pituitary tumor. Acromegaly usually affects middle-aged adults but can cause gigantism in growing children. In adults physical changes usually occur gradually, so the diagnosis may not be made for a long time.

I saw some other patients in the clinic, and Dr. Hunt grabbed me to see another patient with him.

"I've got a patient with methemoglobinemia," he said.

"A Kentucky blue person!" I said. I remembered learning about Kentucky blue people in biochemistry during my first year of medical school.

"Well, he's just a little blue."

We entered the room. The patient was sitting in a chair next to the computer desk. He appeared to be in his late 20s or early 30s, and he was well-groomed, casually dressed. He was a good-looking guy, except his skin had a blue tinge.

"Paul, this is James." Dr. Hunt sat in front of the computer.

"Nice to meet you, James," Paul said. "Dr. Hunt likes for all the students to see me as I'm a bit of a curiosity."

"You have methemoglobinemia?" I sat in a chair, facing the patient.

"That's what they've told me. Try to say that three times real fast."

I smiled.

He laughed. "What can I answer for you?"

"Have you had to take methylene blue?"

"No."

"Have others in your family had the condition?"

"My Grandma Esther and a great grandfather."

"Which side of the family is Esther on?"

"Ma's. She passed some years ago."

"Okay. And how about your great grandfather?"

"He was on Pa's side."

"Do you have any siblings?"

"I have a brother and sister."

Paul had congenital methemoglobinemia, which he inherited as a rare autosomal recessive blood disease that skips generations. Each of his unaffected parents had one copy of a gene that can cause the enzyme cytochrome b5 methemoglobin reductase to be absent from red blood cells (RBCs). Paul had the disease because he had two copies of the gene. He had abnormally high methemoglobin (oxidized hemoglobin) levels on his RBCs, so the RBCs didn't have as much hemoglobin to carry oxygen to tissues. He appeared cyanotic, but he was otherwise asymptomatic.

Normal methemoglobin levels remain below 1%. Levels of 3–15% can cause slight discoloration of the skin. Levels of 15–20% cause mild cyanosis. Levels of 25–50% can cause headache, dyspnea, lightheadedness or syncope, weakness, confusion, palpitations (abnormal heart pulsation), and chest pain. Levels of 50–70% can cause arrhythmia, delirium, coma, and severe acidosis (acidic blood). IV methylene blue should be administered if methemoglobin levels exceed 30%.

The story of the Kentucky blue people can be traced to Martin Fugate, an orphan from France who settled in Troublesome Creek, near Hazard, Kentucky, in 1820. According to family folklore, he was blue. He married Elizabeth Smith, a pale redhead who carried one copy of the recessive gene. They had seven children, and four of them were reported to be blue. The Fugates were isolated in the valleys and hollows of the Appalachian Mountains, with no railroads and few roads outside the region. Zachariah, one of the blue sons, married his mother's sister. Other Fugates married cousins and families who lived nearby.

In 1960 hematologist Dr. Madison Cawein heard rumors of the blue people while he was working at the University of Kentucky's Lexington Medical Clinic, and he decided to investigate. He recruited Ruth Pendergrass, a nurse at the American Heart Association clinic in Hazard, to help him find the blue people. Ruth had seen a dark blue woman in the county health department on a very cold afternoon. Ruth thought the patient was going to die of a heart attack, but the woman wasn't concerned at all. She just wanted a blood test. She said she was related to the blue Combses who lived in Ball Creek, and she was a sister of one of the Fugate women.

Dr. Cawein was able to obtain some blood samples from blue people for analysis at the University of Kentucky. He determined that they had the deficiency in cytochrome b5 methemoglobin reductase, and he returned to the mountains to treat them with methylene blue. Their skin turned a normal color for the first time in their lives, and their urine was blue, so they concluded that they were literally peeing the blue out their bodies.

Incestuous or consanguineous mates are far more likely than random mates to produce offspring with rare genetic diseases. A person has an average of five to eight recessive, deleterious genes, and siblings share about half of the mutations. Direct relatives are far more likely to share mutations than the rest of the population. Congenital methemoglobinemia has affected six generations, but the blood disorder is rarer today because Appalachian people have dispersed and the family gene pool is much more diverse. Most of the blue Fugates never suffered any health effects and lived into their 80s and 90s.

I left the clinic to go to AVMC. Ms. Thacker was still unable to ambulate, and she was diagnosed with a heart condition. Telemetry showed bradycardia (abnormally slow heart rate) during the night, so Dr. Coleman ordered an EKG while he was on call. The EKG showed a Mobitz type 2 atrioventricular (AV) block, an electrical conduction system problem from the atria to the ventricles. Cardiology was consulted for pacemaker implantation. A CT angiogram was ordered for Ms. Blackburn to visualize her 91-year-old coronary arteries. I also saw Sarah, a 15-year-old female with lupus who was admitted for multilobar pneumonia (infection in two or more lung lobes).

I returned to the clinic to see patients. My Motorola Razr flip phone vibrated. My stepmother was calling.

"Hello," I said.

"James, this is Mary," she said. "Your dad's been in a car accident."

"What happened?"

"His car went off the road and down an embankment in the rain. The car was totaled, but he was wearing his seat belt. He was able to get out and walk up to the road, and another driver stopped and called 911. He had internal bleeding, and he's in surgery now to have his spleen removed."

"I'm sorry, Mary. When did he go into surgery?"

"They just took him back."

"Okay. How was he before surgery?"

"He was in pain and feeling like he was going to pass out, but he still had his sense of humor. Pain medicine made him a little goofy."

"That sounds like Dad. How are you doing?"

"Well, I'm shaken up and worried about him, of course."

"Of course. I'm sorry, Mary. I'm in a clinic now, seeing patients. Could you call me after he's out of surgery?"

"Yes."

"Okay. I'll pray for his surgery to go well."

"Thank you."

"Of course. Love you."

"Love you too."

"Bye."

I shared the bad news with Dr. Coleman. He told me to go see my father, and I told him I wanted to wait to see how he was doing after surgery before planning a trip. I saw a couple of patients and returned home. Mary called me later in the evening to tell me the surgery went well, and Dad was sedated and on a ventilator.

On Friday Dr. Coleman again told me I didn't have to come in for a half day, so I read about pancreatitis (pancreas inflammation). Dad was still on a ventilator.

On Saturday I was glad to be able to talk to my father. "Hi, Dad. How are you doing?"

"I'm okay, son," he said. "Sorry my speech is a little slurred. I think the morphine's too strong. It's making me feel loopy. It's good to hear from you."

"It's good to talk to you too. So you somehow managed to work your breathing tube out without the use of your hands, which were restrained?"

"What can I say? Your old dad's got talent. I wanted that thing out, so I got it out."

"I can't say I'm surprised you did that."

"You know your dad well."

"So your car slid off the road on a curve in the rain?"

"Yeah. And I wasn't going fast. I was actually driving a little below the speed limit."

"How were the tires?"

"They needed to be replaced. I just hadn't done it yet."

"Well, I hope you don't ever let tires get that bad again."

"I know. I will definitely be much better about that from now on."

"Good."

"So how's your clinical experience going? What are you doing now?"

"I'm on a family medicine rotation. It's going well. The doctors are cool, and I've seen quite a few interesting patients."

"Well, good. I'm so proud of my firstborn doctor to be. I brag about you to everyone."

"Thanks, Dad. Any idea how much longer you'll be in the hospital?"

"I'm not sure yet, but I want to get out of here as soon as I can."

"I need to complete another week of this rotation to fulfill my requirement for the month. How about if I come to see you next weekend?"

"That would be wonderful, son."

"Okay. I love you."

"I love you too."

"Bye."

On Monday I returned to AVMC. Ms. Thacker remained bedridden, and she was scheduled for pacemaker placement the next day. Ms. Blackburn had turned 92 over the weekend, and she had been diagnosed with coronary artery disease (CAD) and HTN. Cardiology recommended for her to be treated conservatively with aspirin, simvastatin, metoprolol, and nitroglycerin as needed for chest pain. She was discharged. Sarah received Levaquin (antibiotic) for pneumonia, and she continued to spike fevers.

On Tuesday Ms. Thacker still couldn't ambulate after having her pacemaker placed, and Sarah continued to be febrile. I continued to see them and some other inpatients over the next couple of days, including a 61-year-old female with acute pancreatitis, nausea, and vomiting after she had surgery for a kidney stone; a 56-year-old female with severe COPD and respiratory insufficiency; and an 84-year-old female with CHF.

On Friday Lynn and I made the eight-hour drive to West Tennessee to visit my father and Mary for the weekend. Dad was home in good spirits and functioning well, but he had rib and hip pain and difficulty taking full breaths. I did an osteopathic exam, and I determined that a left rib was stuck in an exhaled position, and his medial ankles were uneven due to a hip shear.

I performed OMT, and he was very pleased with the result. Pain was much better, and he was able to breathe and walk normally.

Lynn and I returned to Brighton on Monday, and I resumed my rotation in Branham on Tuesday. Ms. Thacker and Sarah were no longer in AVMC. I continued my rotation through September, and I saw plenty of other interesting cases. At the end of the rotation, Dr. Coleman gave me a glowing evaluation, and I thanked him for the experience. I would miss him and Dr. Hunt.

Endnotes

1. Erythematous: abnormal redness due to inflammation or infection.

2. Edematous: abnormally swollen with fluid.

3. Suboxone (buprenorphine/naloxone) is FDA-approved for treatment of opioid dependence. Buprenorphine is a partial mu opioid agonist, unlike other opioids, which are full mu opioid agonists. Buprenorphine is combined with naloxone (an opioid antagonist) to deter intravenous (IV) use. Naloxone is poorly absorbed when taken orally but has good bioavailability when injected. A buprenorphine overdose has a very low risk for causing lethal respiratory depression, unless the patient's health is compromised, or the medication is combined with another central nervous system depressant, such as a benzodiazepine (especially with IV use). Buprenorphine also has a higher affinity for mu opioid receptors than full mu opioid agonists, so it prevents the other opioids from binding to the mu receptors and reduces the risk of the patient dying of an OxyContin or heroin overdose.

4. Subutex (buprenorphine) is recommended for opioid-dependent pregnant patients to avoid the risk of IV Suboxone use precipitating opioid withdrawal and causing fetal distress.

5. "Percs, Roxis, Oxys": Percocet, Roxicodone (oxycodone), OxyContin (extended-release oxycodone).

6. Coreg (carvedilol) is a beta blocker that is used to decrease blood pressure and heart rate. The medication also blocks alpha adrenergic (adrenaline) receptors, like labetalol. Other beta blockers affect only beta receptors.

7. Metanephrine: breakdown product of epinephrine (adrenaline). Catecholamines: epinephrine, norepinephrine, dopamine. Vanillylmandelic acid: breakdown product of catecholamines.

8. Colostomy: a surgically created connection between the lumen of the colon and an opening in the abdominal wall.

9. Chronic obstructive pulmonary disease (COPD) is usually caused by a combination of emphysema (destruction of alveoli, the lungs' small respiratory sacs) and chronic bronchitis (inflammation of bronchi, the lungs' branching airways).

10. Percocet is an opioid. Zofran is an antinausea medication.

11. Arteriovenous fistula: surgically created communication between an artery and vein.

12. Troponin is a cardiac muscle protein that is elevated in the blood if muscle damage has occurred.

13. A Holter monitor is a battery-operated portable device that records the heart's electrical activity (EKG) continuously for 24–48 hours or longer.

14. Angina pectoris: chest pain.

15. Percocet and Lortab are opioids, and tramadol is a mild opioid that also increases the levels of neurotransmitters serotonin and norepinephrine, like antidepressants.

16. Neurontin (gabapentin) is an antiepileptic that is FDA-approved for partial seizures and postherpetic neuralgia, and the medication is used off-label for chronic pain and anxiety. Lyrica (pregabalin) is an antiepileptic that is FDA-approved for neuropathic pain, postherpetic neuralgia, fibromyalgia, and partial seizures as adjunct treatment. Gabapentin has become a drug of abuse, but the DEA hasn't designated it as a controlled substance, even though it is very similar to Lyrica, which is a controlled substance. Kentucky was the first state to classify gabapentin as a Schedule V medication in 2017. Since then Alabama,

Michigan, North Dakota, Tennessee, Virginia, and West Virginia have followed suit, and 12 other states have required reporting of gabapentin to their controlled substance monitoring programs. The FDA issued a warning 12/19/19 about the risk of "serious breathing difficulties" in patients using gabapentin or pregabalin with opioids or other central nervous system depressants, as well as those with respiratory conditions and the elderly.

17. Lisinopril, metformin, and simvastatin are used to treat HTN, DM, and hyperlipidemia (HLD), respectively.

18. HbA1c is a lab that measures an average blood glucose level over the past 3 months.

Chapter 4

Osteopathic Medicine

I started my OMT rotation with Richard Metz, D.O., at the beginning of October. I arrived at Brighton Medical Center (BMC), a 266-bed hospital, at 7:50 a.m. Dr. Metz's office was in the family medicine clinic on the second floor. I parked my nine-year-old Volvo sedan near some exotic cars in the physicians' parking area, and I peeked at the beautiful interior of a Maserati GranTurismo on my way to the clinic. Dr. Metz was a professor of osteopathic principles and practice (OPP) at BCSOM and director of neuromusculoskeletal medicine at BMC. He had a reputation as an OMT guru. He lectured around the country for other medical schools and hospitals.

His office door was open, and he was sitting at his desk, checking email on his desktop computer. He appeared older, trim, with receded gray-and-white hair, and a beard, wearing glasses, a light yellow Oxford shirt, and khaki pants. Stacks of patient charts in manila folders were on his desk. His office was dim because his overhead fluorescent lights were off and there was no desk lamp. Overcast morning light was coming through the blind of his window. Classical music was quietly playing from his computer speakers.

"Dr. Metz. Good morning," I said. "I'm James Banks. I'm supposed to start my OMT rotation today."

He stood and shook my hand. "Nice to meet you, James."

"Nice to meet you."

"Have a seat. What other rotations have you done so far?"

"Just family medicine." I sat in a chair next to his desk.

He smiled. "Well, that's a great rotation to start with. A lot of D.O.s go into primary care, and they make great family docs. Where are you from?"

"Tennessee."

"Tennessee's a pretty state. I've been to Nashville and Knoxville."

"I grew up in a small town between Memphis and Nashville, and I have some college friends in Nashville, but I like the eastern part of the state better. I like the mountains. Where are you from?"

"I'm originally from Wisconsin, but I haven't lived there since I graduated college. I went to medical school in Chicago, then jobs took me to other places."

"What brought you here?"

"I had an opportunity to be chair of the OPP department of a brand-new osteopathic school, so I started here in 1996 when BCSOM was founded."

"Cool. So how do you and your wife like Brighton?"

"Well, our house is in Lexington. I stay in an apartment here during the week, and I spend weekends in Lexington. Brighton's a pretty neat town. Are you familiar with tensegrity?"

"No, I'm not sure if I've ever heard of the term."

"What about Hygeian versus Asclepian medicine?"

"No, I'm not familiar with those terms either."

"Well then, we should talk about how tensegrity and Hygeian and Asclepian medical philosophies relate to osteopathic medicine."

He opened a PowerPoint presentation on his computer screen, titled, "Brighton Medical Center, Osteopathic Principles and Practice." He clicked to the next slide, which was titled, "A.T. Still, M.D, D.O. 1952 Tenets from the Kirksville College of Osteopathy and Surgery." He read the tenets: "The body is a functional unit. Structure and function are reciprocally interrelated. The body is a self-regulating system; the body makes its own medicines. Rational treatment should be based on these principles." The slide had two portraits of Dr. Still.

He clicked to the next slide, which was titled "Where I'm coming from!" He said, "So if we apply these tenets to illness, we have a paradigm of host plus disease equals illness."

He clicked to the next slide, which was dense with many words in four different colors. He said, "To better understand this paradigm, we have to consider the history of medicine and the Hygeian and Asclepian philosophies. The Hygeian school is the host model, and the Asclepian school is the disease model. Let's consider the Hygeian school first.

"Hippocrates viewed health as the *natural state* of the body. He believed the body to endowed with *vis medicatrix naturae*, inherent healing power. The Latin phrase literally means: the healing power of nature.

"Disease is viewed as the *total body's response* to adapt to a new situation or restore health. The origin of disease is *enormously complex*. The goal for a Hygeian physician is to help the patient live within the laws of nature and remove impediments to any of the mechanisms that maintain and restore health.

"The Hygeian philosophy emphasizes personal responsibility. The human body has a vast inventory of endogenous medicines that are an integral component of the body's built-in health-care system. These endogenous medicines are called autocoids.

"Now let's consider Asclepian medicine. The Asclepian school is the major school today. Asclepian medicine focuses on disease and the causes and cures of disease. Disease is viewed as the effect of or response to a specific cause or agent. The disease primarily affects a selected tissue, organ, or system. For each disease, there is presumed to be a chemical agent or modality, which combats either the causative agent, the disease itself, or the symptoms.

"The successful Asclepian physician is one who makes a correct diagnosis and prescribes or administers the effective treatment, so there is a major focus on intervention—especially of a chemical nature. This focus on chemical intervention is enhanced by the germ theory.

"Now let's consider epidemiology from an osteopathic perspective. If the host has lowered resistance to disease due to somatic dysfunction, susceptibility to disease is increased. Environment can also contribute to allostasis and allostatic load, which typically is a strain on the system for at least two to three years."

"What is allostasis?" I said. "I remember it being mentioned in an OMT lecture, but I can't remember what it means."

"Well, allostasis could be a whole other lecture," he said. "Allostasis is an altered state of homeostasis that occurs in response to any stress that threatens homeostasis. The stress can be internal or external to the host. Allostasis allows survival of the host for the short term, but if allostasis persists and becomes chronic, it becomes pathologic, and we refer to it as allostatic load. An allostatic load causes cumulative damage in organ systems, disease, and illness.

"If host plus disease equals illness, we have three different possibilities for this paradigm. Disease can be the primary cause of illness. A problem with the host can be the primary cause of illness. Or host and disease can contribute to illness.

"If disease is the primary cause of illness, allopathic treatment can be very effective. If a problem with the host is the primary cause of illness, osteopathic treatment is more effective. If host and disease contribute to illness, a combination of allopathic and osteopathic treatment is most effective. Even if disease is the primary problem, the best allopathic care can still have disease model failures. We've had plenty of OMT consults for inpatients here who received great medical care but remained stuck in the recovery process. With OMT we helped them recover faster and even use less medication."

He clicked to the next slide. "Kirkaldy-Willis was an internationally recognized M.D. orthopod with 50 years of clinical experience. He coauthored the book *Orthodox and Complementary Medicine*, and he likened the relationship between orthodox disease-oriented medicine and complementary host-oriented medicine to the bond between Newtonian and quantum physics. Clinical work should combine the two approaches because most clinical problems are part Newtonian and part quantum. He recently wrote that effective patient care must address not only a physical diagnosis but also the needs of the *human being* in the context of family, home, work, interests, and spiritual beliefs.

"Now we come to tensegrity, which is an engineering concept. Are you familiar with Donald Ingber?"

"No." I only remembered that one of my classmates said Dr. Metz was "gay for Ingber" because he referenced him a lot.

"Well, he is an M.D., Ph.D., pathologist at Harvard Medical School, and he has studied how mechanical forces through a tensegrity system can actually affect biochemical processes at the cellular level. This is called mechanotransduction, and it's pretty cool. Take a look at this image." The slide had a photo of a tower of connected rods, resembling a radio tower. "None of these rods are touching each other. They are held together with continuous tension wires. And the tower is self-supporting. In fact, you could even say that it defies gravity. It has both structure and function.

"The human body is a tensegrity system. Our bones are like the rods in this tower, and our muscles and fascia are like the wires.

"Here are some key points about tensegrity. We can also consider these to be host truths. A tensegrity system can be a very flexible and lightweight structure. It can have omnidirectional motion potential. Weak materials become stronger than one would predict. Evenly distributed forces instantly travel throughout the system, and the whole system simultaneously adapts to introduced forces.

"The system protects the weakest link just as the human body protects the area of greatest restriction by making compensations. The area of greatest restriction is the greatest hindrance or most dysfunctional part of the system. A change in tissue shape can alter structure and function, biochemical expression, genetic expression. The genetic expression can be health-promoting or disease-promoting. Normal cell shape can promote cell maturation and specialization, while abnormal cell shape can promote uncontrolled cell growth, cancer, and apoptosis" (programmed cell death).

Dr. Metz lectured for what seemed like hours. His slides were dense, packed with images, diagrams, and many words in four different colors. His lecture was interesting, and it stretched my mind, but I wanted to see patients. I struggled to continue to act interested after a while, and I couldn't daydream or doze off because I wasn't in the back of a classroom with other students; I was sitting right next to Dr. Metz in his dim office, which I found depressing. Why didn't he at least have a light on? Overcast morning light coming through the blind of his window was not enough. I started to pay attention again near the end of his lecture when he finally seemed to get to his main point.

"So when we conduct an osteopathic exam on a patient, we look for the area of greatest restriction, and we sequence. A patient may have a headache, but their AGR is in their right ankle. We treat the AGR, and we examine the patient again to see what changes we have made. We then treat the next AGR."

"Okay."

"Treating the AGR and sequencing can be very effective and efficient because the human body is a tensegrity system." He illustrated this point with several actual cases, and he saved the best case for last.

"Now this was a really neat case. We got a great result with this patient. She was a 57-year-old female hospitalized with congestive heart failure, COPD, and parkinsonism. Her internist had adjusted her medications but not added any new ones, and he was hoping to discharge her in three days. An OMT consult was requested on the fourth day, and OMT was started. We treated rib cage dysfunction first, followed by cervical, thoracic, and right upper extremity dysfunction."

He clicked to the next slide, which showed the patient's pulmonary function tests on day of admission, three days later, and six days later. "Check out these numbers on her PFTs. With good allopathic care, her FVC only increased from 27 to 31 percent in three days, her PEF actually decreased from 50.4 to 38.7 percent, and her FEV_1 increased from 24.3 to 34.8 percent. She then received good osteopathic care on days four and five, and her FVC increased to 71 percent, PEF increased to 59 percent, and FEV_1 increased to 80 percent."

"Wow. That's impressive."

"Indeed. Pretty cool, huh?"

I was thankful to finally get to see some patients after a while. I didn't get much hands-on experience because resident Heather Gibson, D.O., was eager to treat all of the patients herself. She planned to incorporate OMT into her family medicine practice. She was cute and slim, wearing purple scrubs and a white lab coat. She presented her exam findings to Dr. Metz, and he conducted his own exam to see if he agreed with the location of the AGR. I was sometimes allowed to touch the patients to see if I could feel the somatic dysfunctions. I had OMT experience from my first two years of medical school, and I thought my skills were reasonable, but I was always intimidated by diagnosing very specific dysfunctions. Effective OMT required highly refined palpation skills, and it appeared as if the skills of Drs. Gibson and Metz were far superior to mine.

One of the patients was Jeffrey Hughes, M.D., a 35-year-old internist who worked in BMC. He had chronic headaches, neck and back pain since he injured himself seven years earlier by falling 40 feet and landing on his left side after a roof collapsed. He would have been a doctor at the time, so I wondered what he was doing on a roof. Dr. Gibson and I saw him in a clinic room. He was sitting on an OMT table, and his white lab coat was draped over a chair. His neck and back were hunched, and he looked very uncomfortable. He appeared young, thin, and nerdy, with short, light brown hair. He was clean-shaven, wearing glasses, a light blue Oxford shirt, and gray pants.

"Hello, Dr. Hughes," Dr. Gibson said. "This is James."

"Nice to meet you," I said.

"Hello." He winced as he strained to raise his neck to make eye contact.

"So you fell through a roof?" I said.

"Yeah," he said. "I was trying to patch up a barn."

"40 feet is a long way to fall," I said.

"It sure is. After that happened, I decided to stick to just being a doctor."

"Doctors shouldn't be on roofs," Dr. Gibson said with a grin. Then she frowned. "Well, you don't look so good today."

"That's why I'm here," he said. "I really need a tune-up."

"I don't see how you can work in that condition."

"It's not easy. My head is pounding, and my back and neck are killing me." He had rated his pain as 10/10.

"Well, let's see what's going on here. Could you stand up for me?" He slowly and painfully stood in front of the table, and Dr. Gibson precisely touched each of his acromioclavicular joints at the same time to check for asymmetry. "Your left shoulder is a little lower than your right." She palpated the anterior superior iliac spines of his hips to check for asymmetry. She placed her thumbs on the posterior superior iliac spines (PSISs) above his buttocks. "Okay, now walk to the door." She kept her thumbs in position, and she walked behind him to check for restriction in pelvic movement. "Okay. You can sit back on the table."

She placed her thumbs on his PSISs again. "Now bend over." She checked for restriction in pelvic movement. "Okay." He straightened his back as much as he could, she palpated his spine, and she narrowed her focus to specific lumbar, thoracic, and cervical vertebrae. She palpated the transverse processes of the vertebrae with her thumbs as she asked him to bend forward and backward. She palpated his flexed forearms to check for restriction to supination or pronation, his legs to check for restriction to external or internal rotation, and his ankles to check for restriction to inversion or eversion. "Okay. Lie on your back." She palpated his ribs while he was breathing normally. "Take some deep breaths." She checked for restrictions in rib movement. "Okay. You can sit up." She wrote her exam findings in his paper chart. "James, could you please ask Dr. Metz to come in?"

I brought Dr. Metz into the room.

"Hello, Jeff," Dr. Metz said. "You don't look so good."

"I don't feel so good," Dr. Hughes said.

"How are the patients treating you?"

"They're wearing me out. I'm thinking about going into cardiology so I can just focus on the heart."

"I understand." Dr. Metz examined him. "Okay. Dr. Gibson, what did you find?"

She replied with her sequenced list of somatic dysfunctions, starting with the AGR: "Right rib 10 restricted, C5 FRS left, L3 FRS left and ERS left, T1 FRS left, left radius and carpals restricted."

I noted the diagnoses in my pocket notebook for my patient log. C5, L3 and T1 refer to cervical, lumbar, and thoracic vertebrae. FRS and ERS are abbreviations for flexed rotated side-bent and extended rotated side-bent, respectively.

"So you want to start with the rib?" Dr. Metz said.

"Yes," Dr. Gibson said.

"Sounds like a plan." He turned to Dr. Hughes. "Good to see you, Jeff. She'll get you fixed up."

"Thanks," Dr. Hughes said.

Dr. Metz left the room.

Dr. Gibson turned to Dr. Hughes. "Okay. Lie on your back." She treated the right 10th rib with balanced ligamentous tension, a technique that is both indirect (away from restrictive barrier) and direct (toward restrictive barrier). She placed light pressure on the rib for a minute or two to hold it at a balance point as he breathed normally. "Okay. Take a deep breath." She palpated the rib to see if it was moving better. "And again." He took another deep breath. "You can sit back up."

She examined his spine again as she had done before, and she decided to treat C5 next. The vertebra was flexed rotated side-bent left, which meant that it was restricted from extending, rotating, and side bending right. She treated C5 with functional technique, which is indirect. She placed her left hand on his head to flex, rotate, and side bend his neck to the left to place C5 in a position of ease, away from the restrictive barrier, as she palpated the transverse processes with the index and middle fingers of her right hand. She held the position for a minute or two then extended and flexed his head to see if the dysfunction was resolved. It is hypothesized that functional technique works by normalizing afferent nerve signal overload to the area and activating the body's intrinsic self-correcting mechanisms.

She examined his thoracic and lumbar spine again, and she decided to treat L3 next.

"You're treating L3 now?" I said.

"Yes," she said.

"And L3 is FRS left and ERS left?"

"Well, now it's just ERS left."

"I didn't know that a vertebra could have flexed and extended dysfunctions at the same time."

"I didn't either until I worked with Dr. Metz. He's awesome."

"That's what I heard. That's why I requested to do my OMT rotation with him."

She treated L3 with functional technique. She placed her right hand on his right shoulder to extend, rotate, and side bend his back to the left to place L3 in a position of ease as she palpated the transverse processes. She held the position for a moment, then she treated T1 and his left wrist with the same technique. "Okay. That's it. How would you rate your pain now?"

"Two. And my headache's gone." His back and neck were now straight, and he appeared relaxed, relieved.

"Great. So you've had an 80 percent reduction in pain, and your headache's gone."

"Wow," I said. "That's impressive."

"She has magic hands," he said. "Thank you, Dr. Gibson. I feel like a new man."

"You're welcome," she said. "I'd like to see you back in two weeks."

"Sounds good."

On the second day of my rotation, we saw a 48-year-old, obese female who had been admitted to PMC for cholecystitis (gallbladder inflammation), and her surgeon requested an OMT consult to see if she could be discharged without surgery and follow up as an outpatient. She also had right forearm pain and restricted movement since she fell and injured her wrist six months earlier. Physical therapy had limited benefit, so she had wrist cartilage reduction surgery five months after the injury, and she felt like the surgery didn't help at all. Dr. Gibson and Dr. Metz examined her, and Dr. Gibson treated the somatic dysfunctions:

1. Dx: AA RR (atlantoaxial joint rotated right, which restricted head from turning left)
   Tx: FCT (functional technique)
2. Dx: C4 FRS_R
   Tx: FCT

3. Dx: Petrous-occipital (cranial fissure) R restriction
   Tx: CS (craniosacral therapy)
4. Dx: T9 ERS$_R$
   Tx: FCT
5. Dx: R ribs 6–10 inhaled
   Tx: MET (muscle energy technique)
6. Dx: R radius pronated
   Tx: MET
7. Dx: R carpals restricted
   Tx: FCT

Muscle energy is a direct technique that involves the patient using active muscle force against the doctor's unyielding counterforce. I'll discuss craniosacral therapy shortly with another interesting case. After Dr. Gibson completed the treatment, the patient had nearly full range of motion of her radius, and she was discharged on the same day with a plan to follow up with her surgeon as an outpatient.

On the third day of my rotation, I saw another hospitalized patient with a different resident, Kimberly Miller, D.O. She was cute and slim, wearing a blouse, pants, and white lab coat. She was as eager as Dr. Gibson to perform OMT on patients. The patient was a 47-year-old female who wasn't passing gas after a hysterectomy, and she had right shoulder and neck pain.

Dr. Miller and Dr. Metz examined her, and Dr. Miller treated the somatic dysfunctions:

1. Dx: AA R$_R$
   Tx: MET
2. Dx: OA ES$_R$R$_L$
   Tx: MET
3. Dx: C4 FRS$_L$
   Tx: MET

4. Dx: R shoulder restricted
   Tx: FCT
5. Dx: R radius pronated
   Tx: MET
6. Dx: T12 FRS$_R$
   Tx: FCT

We followed up with her the next day. She had a good bowel movement in the morning, and shoulder and neck pain had improved. She complained of low back pain, and her right arm was sore.

Dr. Miller treated different somatic dysfunctions:

1. Dx: L3 FRS$_R$
   Tx: FCT
2. Dx: L ribs 1–5 inhaled
   Tx: FCT, MET
3. Dx: T5 FRS$_L$
   Tx: MET

Later that day I saw a head case in the clinic with Scott Walker, D.O. Dr. Walker had completed a family medicine residency, and he was doing a one-year OMT fellowship. The patient was a 60-year-old male who had frequent moderate to severe headaches for the past five months. He had been injured in a mining accident 20 years earlier. A large rock struck the top of his helmet, cracked the helmet, and pushed it over his ears.

Dr. Walker confirmed his diagnosis with Dr. Metz:

1. L1 ERS$_L$
2. Petrous-occipital R
3. Frontal lesser wing B/L (bilateral)
4. Petrous-sphenoid R

5. Spheno-squamous L

6. SBS (sphenobasilar synchondrosis) L shear

Cranial osteopathy/craniosacral treatment originated with William Sutherland, D.O., in the 1930s. He graduated from the American School of Osteopathy, and he was an early student of A.T. Still. He claimed that the individual bones of the skull are mobile, and he proposed that the cranial bones, sacrum, dural membranes, central nervous system (CNS), and cerebrospinal fluid (CSF) functioned as a moving unit, which he named the primary respiratory mechanism (PRM). The dura mater is a tough, fibrous membrane that surrounds the CNS, and it attaches to the sacrum. Dr. Sutherland also claimed that rhythmic impulses could be palpated through the skull. This was later called the cranial rhythmic impulse (CRI), which is caused by the CSF circulating with a pulse of 10–14 cycles per minute. Craniosacral therapy involves gentle pressure to somatic dysfunctions of the head and other parts of the body to manipulate the PRM/CRI.

Craniosacral therapy has poor scientific evidence to support its use, however, so it has received "widespread and vigorous critical attention compared with other fields of osteopathic medicine," according to "Therapeutic Effects of Cranial Osteopathic Manipulative Medicine: A Systematic Review," published in the *Journal of the American Osteopathic Association* in December 2011. The meta-analysis examined seven randomized controlled trials and one observational study and concluded, "the currently available evidence on the clinical efficacy of cranial OMM is heterogeneous and insufficient to draw definitive conclusions. Because of the moderate methodological quality of the studies and scarcity of available data, further research into this area is needed."

According to "Cranial Osteopathy: Its Fate Seems Clear," published in *Chiropractic and Osteopathy* in June 2006, "This treatment regime lacks a biologically plausible mechanism, shows no diagnostic reliability, and offers little hope that any direct clinical effect will ever be shown. In spite of almost uniformly negative research findings, 'cranial' methods remain popular with many practitioners and patients. Until outcome studies show that these techniques produce a direct and positive clinical effect, they should be dropped from all academic curricula; insurance companies should stop paying for them; and patients should invest their time, money, and health elsewhere."

Dr. Walker treated the patient's L1 with FCT and the cranial dysfunctions with gentle pressure from his fingers. Craniosacral therapy was intriguing and mysterious to me. I was allowed to do some palpation, and I felt some subtle differences between bilateral sutures, where bones met, but I wasn't sure if I felt the CRI. Despite craniosacral therapy being questionable, Dr. Walker's treatment was effective. The patient's headache resolved.

I saw several coal miners in the clinic on other days. One was a 38-year-old male with chronic low back pain and leg radiculopathy—pain, numbness, or weakness from nerve root injury or irritation—after a Mack truck tailgate fractured his back in two places eight years earlier, and he later had back surgery. He complained of groin pain and numbness and tingling in his left leg. Caudal and facet injections offered some relief, but one physical therapy session worsened his symptoms, so he didn't return for PT. He also had lumbar degenerative disc disease.

Another 46-year-old miner complained of bilateral hip and leg pain, burning and tingling in his right foot. He had been injured in a mining accident six years earlier. A large rock fell on the back of his legs and fractured his right medial and lateral ankle. Another 58-year-old male had been a miner for 30 years, and he complained of low back pain, neck pain, a sore left rib, and burning pain below both knees. All of the miners benefited from OMT.

One day I saw a patient with only Dr. Metz, who had been consulted after the patient was treated by a resident. He was a 48-year-old male with only one somatic dysfunction: L5 FRS_L. Dr. Metz treated him with FCT, and his blood pressure dropped from 139/92 to 124/85.

On another day I saw four interesting cases. One was a 62-year-old female with neck and shoulder pain. She had been in a motor vehicle accident (MVA) at age 8; her upper body went through the windshield, her teeth went through her lower lip, and she required plastic surgery. At age 56 she was diagnosed with dermatomyositis, a progressive condition with a skin rash, muscle inflammation, and weakness. She previously had chronic headaches and sinusitis, she was on 12 doses of methotrexate (MTX, a rheumatologic medication) per week, and muscle weakness prevented her from participating in family activities. She had started yoga six years earlier, a keto diet three years earlier, and OMT two and a half years earlier. She had been off MTX for two years, and she was able to participate in family activities.

A 28-year-old pregnant female had a 37-week-old fetus in a breech presentation (buttocks or feet down) that was corrected with OMT so she would be able to avoid a C-section as long as the baby behaved itself and stayed in a vertex position (head down).

A 46-year-old female had an impressive 12 somatic dysfunctions, so she *really* needed OMT. She complained of neck pain with arm radiculopathy, headache, low back pain, and bilateral radiculopathy to the toes (tingling, sometimes numbness of the right leg). She had been in remission from malignant melanoma for six years, her C4/5 and C5/6 discs were herniated, her ribs had been broken in high school, she had been in an MVA 12 years earlier, boxes fell on her right shoulder at work 10 years earlier, both her ankles had been sprained, and she had fluid removed from her right knee.

A 62-year-old male had been struck by lightning 25 years earlier, and both his arms were burned. He fractured his coccyx 16 years earlier when he fell off a bulldozer. He had surgery for resection of stomach cancer three years earlier, and he subsequently had multiple abdominal hernias. I thought he was an interesting case because he had survived a lightning strike!

Observing residents treat patients with OMT soon became about as interesting as watching grass grow. Thankfully, I got to treat some patients myself in BCSOM's OMT clinic once or twice a week, and members of my family appreciated me treating their aches and pains. I relieved my wife's chronic back and neck pain and headaches. She had Scheuermann's kyphosis (hunchback) like her father, so she was prone to chronic problems. Her father was 70, so his kyphosis was severe, and I was able to loosen him up so he could straighten his back a little. I relieved my stepmother's sinus congestion.

By the end of October, I was looking forward to starting my general surgery rotation. The autumn air started to turn crisp. The sun's arc was a little lower, and shadows grew longer. The Appalachian Mountains turned into a beautiful mosaic of red, orange, yellow, and green. Dr. Metz gave me a good evaluation, and I thanked him for the experience.

Chapter 5

General Surgery

I started my two-month surgery rotation with Mark Davis, D.O., at the beginning of November. Brighton was in a small valley, and shadows darkened the town before 5 p.m. when the sun set behind the mountains. I was apprehensive about starting the rotation, but I expected it to be interesting. Dr. Davis was also a graduate of BCSOM's first class in 2000, like Drs. Coleman and Hunt. He had been practicing for three years since he completed a grueling, five-year residency to become a general surgeon. Residencies for family medicine, internal medicine, pediatrics, and emergency medicine are three years.

In 2003 the American Council for Graduate Medical Education (the organization that accredits residency programs) implemented restrictions to limit resident physician duty hours to less than 80 per week. Surgical residents, however, commonly work more than 80 hours per week—for five years—but they don't report duty hour violations because they're supposed to be tough and they want their residencies to stay accredited. Surgical residents have fallen asleep standing up while rounding on patients and even in the operating room (OR).

The surgery clinic was five miles from BMC. It was in a single-story medical office building that Dr. Davis shared with other surgeons. I arrived at the front desk on Monday at 8 a.m. to meet him, and a female receptionist took me to the break room.

Dr. Davis was standing next to the coffee maker. He appeared young, overweight, wearing glasses, a blue Oxford shirt, and tan pants. He was eating a donut with one hand and holding a cup of coffee with his other hand.

"Dr. Davis. Good morning," I said. "I'm James Banks. I'm supposed to start my surgery rotation with you."

"Hi, James," he said. "Man, you're tall. Want a donut?"

"No thanks."

"Coffee?"

"I'm good, thanks. I had a cup of coffee before I left my apartment."

"Okay. What rotations have you done so far?"

"OMT and family medicine."

"Have you decided on a specialty?"

"Psychiatry, I think."

"Seriously!"

"Yeah, as long as I like my psych rotation."

"So you don't want to be a real doctor?"

"I guess not."

"I'm just kidding with you, man." He smiled, finished his donut with a big bite, and took a sip of coffee. "I'm tired. I was on call last night, and I had to do an appy.[1] Why don't you go see all the patients and tell me how they're doing?"

"Okay. Do you have a patient list?" I tensed up.

"Yeah, but it's your first day, and I've been asked to go easier on medical students." He didn't smile. "We'll see them together. I hate clinic. I'd rather be in the OR."

"Okay." My anxiety worsened.

We went to see the first patient, a 65-year-old female in an exam room. She was following up to discuss the result of a surgical breast biopsy. She appeared her stated age, well-groomed, wearing a blue paper drape over her torso, sitting on an exam table.

"Ms. Maynard. Hello," Dr. Davis said. "This is James. He's a medical student working with me."

"Hi," I said.

"Nice to meet you," she said.

"How are you?" he said to her.

"Well, I'm nervous about how my test turned out," she said.

"Of course. Well, I've got good news. Your breast biopsy didn't show cancer. It showed what we call ductal hyperplasia. That means your ducts have more cells than normal, but the cells aren't atypical, so you don't need surgery."

"Well, that is good news."

"Yes. I need to take a look at your incision."

"Okay."

Dr. Davis lifted the drape and examined a small, healing incision on her left breast. "It looks good." He lowered the drape. "You don't have to schedule a follow-up with me. You can see me again if you need to. You're a nice lady, but I hope I don't have to see you again. You can follow up with your primary care doctor."

"Okay. Thank you, Dr. Davis."

"You're welcome. Take care."

Dr. Davis and I left the room and went to see the next patient, an 81-year-old female who was following up to discuss the result of an EGD.[2] She appeared her stated age, casually dressed, sitting in a chair. Her grayish white hair was messy but clean.

"Ms. Damron. Hello," Dr. Davis said. "This is James. He's a medical student."

"Hi, James," she said.

"Nice to meet you," I said.

"How are you?" Dr. Davis sat on a rolling stool in front of her.

"Fair to middlin'," she said.

"Okay. Your EGD showed gastritis but no ulcers. That means your stomach is irritated and inflamed. You should avoid booze and Aleve, which can cause gastritis."

"I don't drink! I'm a Christian."

Dr. Davis smiled. "Well, good. You can take Tylenol, instead of Aleve. Keep taking your omeprazole to protect your stomach, and you should avoid spicy foods."

"Okay."

"You can follow up with your primary care doctor."

"Okay. Thank you."

"You're welcome. Take care."

Dr. Davis and I left the room and went to see the next patient, a 38-year-old female who was following up for a cholecystectomy.[3] She appeared older than her stated age, obese, casually dressed, sitting on an exam table.

"Ms. Ratliff. Hello," Dr. Davis said. "This is James. He's a medical student."

"Hi, James," she said.

"Nice to meet you," I said.

"How are you doing?" Dr. Davis said to her.

"Well, I've had some upset stomach, heartburn, and diarrhea," she said.

"Have you had any nausea or vomiting?"

"I've had some nausea, but it's not nearly as bad as it was before."

"Good. Sometimes the stomach and bowel can get irritated after the gallbladder is removed. James, what's this syndrome called?"

"I don't know," I said.

"Sounds like you need to do some reading tonight," he said.

"Sure," I said.

He turned back to the patient. "Hopefully, your symptoms will settle down in a little while. Keep taking your Nexium for your stomach. I need to look at your incisions."

"Okay." She lifted her shirt, and he examined four small, healing incisions on her abdomen.

"They look good." He lowered her shirt. "I'd like to see you back in a month."

"Okay. Thank you, Dr. Davis."

"You're welcome. I hope you get to feeling better."

Dr. Davis and I left the room and went to see the next patient, a 39-year-old male who was following up for a colostomy and removal of a dialysis catheter from his right internal jugular vein. He appeared his stated age, casually dressed, sitting on an exam table. He had been in an MVA, and blunt abdominal trauma tore his colon and caused internal bleeding and leakage of feces. The catheter had been placed after he developed acute renal (kidney) failure.

"Mr. Adkins. Hello," Dr. Davis said. "This is James."

"Hi," I said.

"Hi, James," Mr. Adkins said.

"How are you?" Dr. Davis said to him.

"I'm glad to have that catheter out, but I sure don't like having to have a bag to collect my shit," Mr. Adkins said.

"I know, but we should be able to close that in a few months."

"I can't wait 'cause this sucks. It's not exactly a turn-on for my girlfriend."

"So she's not kinky?"

"She's not *that* kind of kinky!"

Dr. Davis smiled. "I need to take a look at your stoma."[4]

"Okay." Mr. Adkins smiled and raised his shirt, and Dr. Davis removed the empty colostomy bag to examine the stoma.

"It looks good," Dr. Davis said. "Are you cleaning it after you change your bag?"

"Yes."

"Good." Dr. Davis stuck the colostomy bag back in place, lowered his shirt, and examined the healing incision over the right internal jugular vein. "This looks good too. I'll see you back in two months."

"Okay. Thanks."

"You're welcome."

Dr. Davis and I left the room and went to see the next patient, a 62-year-old female who was following up for a HIDA[5] scan and Mediport[6] placement. She appeared older than her stated age, well-groomed and well-dressed, sitting in a chair. The HIDA scan had been ordered because she had gallstone symptoms (biliary colic,[7] nausea, vomiting), but the ultrasound showed no gallstones. She was planning to receive chemotherapy through the Mediport.

"Ms. Hatfield. Hello," Dr. Davis said. "This is James."

"Hi, James," she said.

"Nice to meet you," I said.

"How are you doing?" Dr. Davis sat on a rolling stool in front of her.

"The pain is still coming and going, and sometimes it's really bad," she said. "It's worse after meals. I vomited the other day."

"Are you avoiding fatty foods?"

"As much as I can, but it's hard to completely avoid fat."

"I know. Well, you don't have gallstones, but your HIDA scan showed a low bile ejection fraction. This means your gallbladder isn't contracting properly to squeeze bile into your small bowel. James, what are Rome III criteria?"

"I don't know," I said.

"James has some learning to do." He smiled at her. "You've had your symptoms for about one month?"

"Yes," she said.

"Treatment experts recommend that symptoms should persist for at least three months before considering surgery."

"I don't know if I can stand this for two more months."

"Okay. Well, I can remove your gallbladder laparoscopically by making four small incisions in your belly, and you should be able to go home the same day or next day as long as everything goes well. If the laparoscopic approach turns out to be too difficult, I'll have to open you up by making a six-inch incision below your right ribs, and you'll be in the hospital for two to three days. You may feel much better after surgery, but some people still have symptoms after surgery. And, of course, there are risks with the surgery, like infection, bleeding, damage to your liver, bile duct, or small bowel."

"If there's a chance I'll feel better, I think I want to have the surgery."

"Okay, but you'll also be having chemotherapy, which can cause nausea, vomiting, and abdominal pain. I need to take a look at your Mediport incision."

"Okay." She raised her shirt, and he examined the healing incision over the port beneath her left clavicle.

"It looks good. I'm sorry you're feeling so bad, but I still recommend you take some more time to think about surgery."

"Okay. Thank you, Dr. Davis."

We saw a few more patients in the clinic, and I returned home to do some reading in *Essentials of General Surgery*, fourth edition, to find answers to Dr. Davis's questions. Lynn happily greeted me when I entered our apartment.

"Hi, babe. How was your day?" she said, smiling.

"Okay," I said. "I just saw patients in the clinic today. I'll be in the hospital tomorrow. You appear to be in a good mood. What are you smiling about?"

"I have some news."

"Okay. What is it?"

"I'm pregnant!"

"Wow! That's great news, babe!"

"I know! I'm so happy! I've wanted this for so long." She was emotional with tears of joy.

"I know. I'm happy too." I embraced her, and we hugged tightly.

"I saw Dr. Border today, and she did an ultrasound. She didn't see anything yet, but I'm only six weeks along."

Lynn was 37 years old, and it had been difficult for her to become pregnant for the first time. We enjoyed sex, but it became more of a duty when we had to schedule sex around the time of her ovulation. Dr. Border did an ultrasound of her ovaries, which showed plenty of eggs, and she prescribed Clomid to increase her chances of becoming pregnant. The medication didn't help, so Lynn stopped it after a few months.

Dr. Border also recommended for my semen to be evaluated, so our family doctor ordered the lab for me. Very early one morning, while it was still dark outside, I quietly got out of bed and tiptoed to our small living room with a specimen cup. I sat at our small desk to view porn on our iMac and summon a semen sample. While I was in the middle of doing the deed, Lynn suddenly appeared in the room and startled me.

"What are you doing!" she said.

"What are you doing up!" I said. "I have to put a fucking sperm sample in this cup and rush it to the hospital." I was angry and embarrassed at the same time.

"At five in the morning?"

"Go back to bed."

She went back to bed. I finished the deed, showered, and rushed the sample to the BMC lab in my pants pocket to keep it warm. A lab tech determined that I had plenty of good swimmers.

On the second day of my surgery rotation, I skipped the 7 a.m. morning report to see Dr. Davis's patients in BMC. As soon as the elevator opened on the fourth (surgical) floor, I noticed the smell of feces. I grabbed the patients' paper chart binders from the nurses' station and went to the rectangular doctors' room, which was adjacent to the nurses' station. The room had long desks with computers on opposite walls, and a few doctors were in the room.

Doctors' illegible progress notes and orders were handwritten in paper charts, and the EMR contained vitals, labs, imaging, dictated reports, and medication lists. I sat in front of a computer, spent some time familiarizing myself with the EMR, and I reviewed the charts. Dr. Davis had nine patients on his list, including patients with pancreatitis, abdominal pain, vomiting, anemia, and pressure ulcers. I wondered why two patients were on his list, including a 69-year-old male with CHF, confusion, bilateral venous stasis (stagnant blood flow); and a 44-year-old male with renal failure and hypokalemia.[8]

I went to see a 35-year-old unemployed female with recurrent acute pancreatitis. She was sitting up in bed, watching TV. She appeared older than her stated age, wearing a hospital gown. She had an IV line connected to a bag of normal saline, and she had an NPO[9] order.

"Ms. Caudill. Hello," I said. "I'm James. I'm a medical student working with Dr. Davis."

"Hi, James," she said.

"You were admitted last night for acute pancreatitis?"

"Yeah. I was partying a little too hard. I shouldn't have been drinking that much."[10]

"How much did you drink?"

"I don't know. I lost count, and the next thing I knew, I was in the hospital."

"What were you drinking?"

"Beer."

"You've had two other episodes of pancreatitis?"

"Yeah. I've been told I shouldn't drink."

"That's right. Pancreatitis can kill you."

"I know. I've learned my lesson this time. I can't ever drink like that again."

"You should actually completely avoid alcohol. This is your third episode of pancreatitis. One beer could cause another episode and kill you."

"I know."

"Okay. How are you feeling?"

"Like shit."

I smiled. "Could you be more specific?"

"My stomach hurts, and I'm nauseous."

"Any vomiting?"

"Not since I've been getting medicine."

"How has the morphine been working for the pain?"

"Thank God for morphine! The pain was really bad before I got the morphine."

"I'm glad the morphine has helped. I need to examine you."

"Sure."

I auscultated her heart, lungs, and abdomen. I gently pressed on the epigastric area of her abdomen just below her breastbone.

"Ow." She winced.

"Sorry," I said. "Dr. Davis will see you this morning."

"Okay. Thanks."

"You're welcome."

I left the room and went to see a 45-year-old disabled female with acute pancreatitis. She was asleep in bed, snoring. She appeared older than her stated age, obese, wearing a hospital gown. She had an IV line connected to a bag of normal saline, and she had an NPO order.

"Ms. Bevins," I said.

She continued to snore.

"Ms. Bevins," I said louder.

She awakened. "Oh, hello."

"Good morning, Ms. Bevins. I'm James. I'm a medical student with Dr. Davis."

"Nice to meet you, James."

"Nice to meet you. You were admitted yesterday for acute pancreatitis?"

"That's what they told me."

"And you were drinking alcohol before this happened?"

"Yeah. I've drank for years, but I've never had anything like this happen before."

"You've never had another episode of pancreatitis?"

"No."

"How much did you drink?"

"Oh, about a pint, I guess."

"A pint of what?"

"Jack Daniels,[11] but I don't drink that much every day."

"You drink every day?"

"No."

"How often do you drink?"

"Oh, I don't know. Maybe every other day."

"How much do you usually drink?"

"About half a pint."

"Okay. How are you feeling?"

"I've been better."

"Any nausea or vomiting?"

"I don't have anything left to throw up, but I've still felt sick to my stomach, and I've had some dry heaves."

"How about pain?"

"The medicine has helped a lot, but the pain is still there."

"Okay. I need to examine you."

"Okay."

I examined her as I did the other patient, and she also had epigastric tenderness.

"Dr. Davis will see you this morning," I said.

"Okay. Thanks," she said.

"You're welcome."

I left the room and saw a few more patients. I did a history and physical for a 74-year-old male with renal failure, multiple pressure ulcers, and septicemia (virulent bacteria and their toxins in the blood). He had the ulcers because he was immobile due to a stroke and he had poor nursing home care. As I was walking down the hall, I saw Dr. Davis standing at the nurses' station, talking to two nurses, and I stopped to talk to him. He was wearing a white Oxford shirt and gray pants.

"Good morning, Dr. Davis," I said. "I still have four more patients to see."

"Top of the morning to you, James. Sounds like you need to get here earlier." He looked at me over the tops of his glasses as he said this, and the nurses smiled.

"I was thinking the same thing."

"Sounds good. Have you seen the patients with pancreatitis?"

"Yes."

"Have you graded the severity of their pancreatitis, according to Ranson's criteria?"

"I'm not familiar with Ranson's criteria, but I did some reading last night to answer the questions you asked me yesterday. The lady with dyspepsia, heartburn, and diarrhea has postcholecystectomy syndrome. Rome III criteria are used to assess patients suspected of having biliary dyskinesia. Criteria include pain episodes that last longer than 30 minutes; severe pain that disrupts daily activity or leads to ED visits; pain that isn't relieved by bowel movements, postural changes, or antacids; nausea, vomiting; recurrent symptoms at variable intervals; exclusion of other structural diseases that could explain the symptoms; normal LFTs,[12] conjugated bilirubin, amylase, lipase."

"Okay. Tonight you can read about Ranson's criteria."

Jerry Bailey, D.O., director of the osteopathic family medicine residency, arrived at the nurses' station. He was neatly dressed with a tie and crisp, white lab coat. "Good morning," he politely said to everyone in his soft voice. "James, how are you doing?"

"Okay. How are you?" I said.

"Good. Are you on your surgery rotation with Dr. Davis?"

"Yes."

"I didn't see you at morning report this morning."

"Yeah. It's my first day, and I was rounding on patients."

"Okay. Well, we expect you to attend morning report unless you're in surgery."

"Okay. I'm planning to arrive earlier from now on to round on patients. Dr. Davis, do we have surgery cases tomorrow?"

"I'll be doing scopes in the morning," Dr. Davis said.

"Okay," I said. I was always thankful to have a reason to miss morning report.

"I hope your rotation goes well," Dr. Bailey said to me. "Have a good day."

"Thanks. You too," I said.

Dr. Davis and I quickly saw all the patients together, and he released me to go home to read about Ranson's criteria. Obama was elected president in the evening, and I visualized Dr. Coleman reacting negatively to the news.

The next day I met Dr. Davis and a nurse in an endoscopy room on the first floor at 6 a.m. They were wearing green scrubs and blue paper gowns, standing next to a table, preparing for a screening colonoscopy for the first patient, a 51-year-old female who wasn't yet in the room. They were doing paperwork, checking equipment, and the nurse prepared IV Versed.[13] She was a cute brunette who appeared to be in her 40s. A vitals monitor and video monitor were next to the table. Pop music was playing from a boombox.

"Good morning," I said.

"How's it going?" Dr. Davis said.

"Okay. Still waking up."

"Jennifer, this is James," he said to the nurse. "Is he tall, or what?"

"Hi, James," she said. "You are pretty tall."

"I am. Nice to meet you." I smiled.

"He wants to be a psychiatrist," Dr. Davis said.

"Really?" she said.

"Yeah," I said.

"Well, my mother-in-law could definitely use your services, and I could probably use your help after working with Dr. Davis."

"Oh, come on," he said. "I'm not that hard to get along with."

"At least you don't throw tantrums like Dr. Hung," she said.

"Is he bad?" I said.

"He's on probation for his behavior," she said.

"Oh. He must have serious anger issues."

"He's been in anger management too."

"And it didn't help?"

"Apparently not."

"Do you have any country music on your iPod?" Dr. Davis asked her.

"Sorry," she said. "I don't like country music."

"I'll have to bring my iPod next time," he said. "Where's the patient? Let's get this show on the road. I like to do scopes, but I don't want to be here all day."

"I'll go see if she's ready." She left the room.

"I read about Ranson's criteria for pancreatitis," I said.

"Okay," Dr. Davis said.

"Poor prognostic factors at admission include age greater than 55, white blood cell count greater than 16, glucose greater than 200, LDH greater than 350, and AST greater than 250. Factors 48 hours after admission include a hematocrit decrease of 10, BUN increase of five, estimated fluid sequestration greater than six liters, and calcium less than eight. Having three criteria indicates severe pancreatitis."

"Okay. What are the complications of severe pancreatitis?"

"Pancreatic necrosis, hemorrhage, infection, systemic inflammatory response syndrome, respiratory insufficiency, hypoxemia,[14] renal failure."

"What's Grey Turner's sign?"

"Flank hematoma."[15]

"How about Cullen's sign?"

"Periumbilical hematoma."

"Sounds like you've been doing your reading like a good student. Tonight you can read about inguinal hernias. We have a hernia repair in the morning."

"Okay."

The nurse and patient walked into the room after a few minutes. The patient appeared her stated age, obese, wearing a hospital gown. She was directed to position herself on the table in the left lateral recumbent position (lying on her left side). The nurse hooked her up to the vitals monitor and injected Versed into her IV line to sedate her. Dr. Davis put on nitrile gloves, inserted the colonoscope tip into the patient's anus with his right hand, and advanced the tip. He held a handle with a head of controls in his left hand, and he used two knobs to steer the tip. Video of the illuminated colon was on the monitor.

"She has diverticulosis[16] of the sigmoid colon," he said. "A polyp in the descending colon." He removed the polyp, which would be examined by a pathologist, and he examined the rest of the colon. "Where am I now?" he asked me.

"Is that the ileocecal valve?"[17] I said.

"It is."

Dr. Davis scoped seven patients. An EGD of a 45-year-old female with anemia showed gastritis and duodenal[18] ulcers. A 72-year-old male with brain cancer had a very large polyp and severe diverticulosis. The polyp was probably cancer that had metastasized to his brain. Dr. Davis let me steer the colonoscope for a moment, but he must have not liked my driving. He quickly took the controls back.

I returned home after the last scope to read about inguinal hernias.

The next day I arrived at the OR men's locker room on the first floor at 7:15 a.m. I was excited and nervous. I removed my clothes, wedding ring, and watch, put on clean, green scrubs, tucked my shirt in, and put on a hat, face mask, and shoe covers. I went to a large sink in the hall to thoroughly scrub myself next to Dr. Davis. I used a new disposable brush and antiseptic soap to scrub my fingernails, fingers, between my fingers, and the fronts and backs of my hands for three minutes. Then I scrubbed my forearms for one minute and rinsed. I held my hands above my elbows at all times so water would roll away from my hands. I kept my hands in the position as I followed Dr. Davis to our OR, and I turned to use my back to push the door open.

"Good morning," Dr. Davis said. "I have a medical student with me. This is James."

"Hi, James," the female scrub tech said. Others in the room also greeted me.

"Good morning," I said.

The scrub tech was sterile, wearing a gown, gloves, mask, and hat. She handed each of us a sterile blue towel. I held the towel lengthwise with my right hand to dry my left hand and forearm with one end. When I dried my forearm, I worked the towel in one direction only, from my wrist to my elbow. Then I grabbed the other end of the towel with my dry, left hand, and I dried my right hand and forearm. I dropped the towel in a linen hamper.

"Man, I'm hungry," Dr. Davis said. "I should have grabbed a sausage biscuit on my way in. We're doing a right open inguinal hernia repair for Jed McCoy, date of birth: two four 58."

"Correct," the female circulating nurse said. "Right open inguinal hernia repair for Jed McCoy, date of birth: two four 58." The nurse was nonsterile.

The scrub tech and nurse assisted Dr. Davis with sterile gowning and gloving, then they assisted me. The scrub tech held the sterile gown open in front of me. I pushed my arms into the sleeves, and she pulled the wristlets onto my hands, leaving only my fingers exposed. The nurse tied the back of the gown. The scrub tech held gloves open. I pushed my hands into the gloves, and she pulled the cuffs of the gloves over the sleeve wristlets. I unfastened ties from the front of the gown. I handed the scrub tech the tie that was attached to the back, and I held the tie attached to the front. I did a whirl to close the back of the gown, and I tied the gown in the front.

"Keep your hands above your waist," the scrub tech said. The gown was not considered sterile below the waist.

The patient was a 50-year-old male. His name, date of birth, procedure, and Dr. Davis's name were written on a whiteboard on a wall. He was lying supine (on his back) on the operating table, with his torso exposed, unconscious from anesthesia, which was being administered by a nurse anesthetist. The nurse prepared Jed's surgical site, his right lower abdominal quadrant. She used Betadine and a sponge to scrub his marked incision line first, then she scrubbed outward in a circular motion. After she reached the periphery of the site, she discarded the sponge and repeated the process with a new sponge. The scrub tech and Dr. Davis placed sterile drapes over the torso and clamped the drapes, leaving only a square area over the surgical site exposed.

"Well, get over here," Dr. Davis said to me. "You can't see from there."

"Okay." I was a few steps away from the sterile field. I moved next to Dr. Davis.

"Time out," Dr. Davis said.

"It's 7:47," the nurse said. "We're doing a right open inguinal hernia repair on Jed McCoy, date of birth: two four 58."

"Okay," Dr. Davis said. He used a scalpel to make a transverse (horizontal) incision, a sterile white towel to dab blood, and electrocautery to stop bleeding. Wisps of smoke and the smell of burning flesh rose into the air. The scrub tech passed instruments to him from a draped tray. He dissected fascia deeper in the wound and placed several clamps on the fascia to retract the edges. He handed me a clamp to hold, and I felt a thrill. I was assisting with surgery for the first time! What a privilege this was! During my first year of medical school, I had the privilege of dissecting a cadaver with three classmates. Living human anatomy was much more colorful than dead human anatomy.

"What's this?" Dr. Davis asked me, touching the anatomy.

"The spermatic cord." I said.

"Yes." He placed a sling around the cord to pull it laterally (to the right side). "And here's the hernia sac lateral to the inferior epigastric vessels. So what kind of hernia is this?"

"Indirect."

"Okay. What's a direct hernia?"

"It occurs medial to the epigastric vessels in Hesselbach's triangle. It's caused by a defect in the transversalis fascia."

"What are the boundaries of Hesselbach's triangle?"

"Inferior epigastric vessels, rectus sheath, inguinal ligament."

"Okay. Let's place him in the Trendelenburg position."

The operating table was tilted so the patient's head was lower than his feet. This allowed gravity to retract the herniated tissue into the abdominal cavity. Dr. Davis cut a small slit in a piece of polypropylene (permanent) mesh to accommodate the spermatic cord, and he sewed the mesh in place over the defect.

"You just contaminated yourself," the scrub tech said to me.

"I'm sorry," I said, startled. I had just scratched my thigh with my left hand without realizing it. My right hand was holding a clamp.

"Don't touch anything," she said.

I froze.

"Come on, James," Dr. Davis said emphatically. "What were you thinking!"

"I'm sorry," I said. "I just had an itch and didn't think about it. This is my first time in the OR. This takes some getting used to."

"Okay. Well, use your noggin from now on." His tone was normal. He apparently wasn't really angry. "You'd have to regown and reglove, but this won't take much longer. Why don't you go see how our patients are doing upstairs?"

"Okay."

The scrub tech grabbed the clamp I was holding, and I stepped away from the sterile field. I removed my gloves, gown, and mask near the door and discarded them. I left the room to see the patients.

Ms. Caudill and Ms. Bevins, the alcoholics with pancreatitis, were still NPO. The 45-year-old female with anemia was on sucralfate and Nexium for duodenal ulcers, which had been diagnosed by Dr. Davis the previous day when she had her EGD. I also saw a 43-year-old female with a small bowel obstruction and a 47-year-old male with a buttocks abscess. He was paralyzed from a 1988 MVA.

We didn't have surgical cases the next day, so I arrived at the surgical floor at 5 a.m. and rushed to see eight patients before the 7 a.m. morning report. Ms. Caudill was able to drink and eat, but Ms. Bevins was still NPO. I saw two more patients with pancreatitis, and a 24-year-old female with hypercalcemia (elevated calcium in the blood), anemia, and abdominal lymphadenopathy (enlarged lymph nodes). She probably had cancer. I felt like I didn't do a thorough job rounding on the patients, but at least I saw them all before morning report.

In U.S. graduate medical education, morning report varies among institutions but generally involves transfer of patient information during shift change and case-oriented teaching for resident physicians and medical students. An attending physician is usually present. Selected patients are discussed for their learning value, and management decisions from the previous night are reviewed. At BMC morning report did not consist of a handoff of patient information. It consisted of medical topics that were presented—usually with PowerPoint slides—by attending physicians, residents, and medical students.

Morning report was held in the small medical library. Resident Dr. Gibson gave a PowerPoint presentation about low back pain (LBP), which is a common problem in primary care practice. I was alert since I had been seeing patients for two hours, and I listened because I found the topic interesting.

Dr. Gibson discussed the etiology of LBP; the anatomy of the lumbosacral spine and associated muscles, ligaments, tendons, and nerves; and treatment, including medications, exercise, physical therapy, OMT, and surgery.

I returned to the surgical floor after morning report, and Dr. Davis and I quickly saw the patients together. He decided that Ms. Caudill could be discharged later in the day if she continued to tolerate food without problems. He advised the 24-year-old female with abdominal lymphadenopathy that an oncology consult had been ordered, and he would wait to see what her oncologist recommended.

We left the surgical floor and went to see eight wound care patients on the first floor. The patients had ulcers on their feet, toes, ankles, and heels. One patient had ulcers on his buttocks and shin, two patients had osteomyelitis (bone infection), and most of the patients had poorly controlled diabetes, which caused the ulcers and impaired healing. Wound care looked depressing and hopeless to me, and I wondered if Dr. Davis liked it as much as clinic. Dr. Davis released me after we saw the patients, and I happily returned home. I had survived the first week of my surgery rotation. Dr. Davis didn't require me to be on call with him, but he told me he'd call me if he had an appendectomy case in the middle of the night.

I enjoyed a relaxing Saturday with Lynn. On Sunday I was on call with a family medicine resident, so I rounded on four inpatients with him. I had previously seen one of the patients with Dr. Davis. The 74-year-old male with renal failure, multiple pressure ulcers, and septicemia had his diagnosis updated to sepsis secondary to polymicrobial pneumonia, and chronic renal failure.

On Monday of my second week, I was happy to skip morning report to observe a "lap chole" (laparascopic cholecystectomy). The patient was Ms. Bevins, the 45-year-old alcoholic female with pancreatitis. Dr. Davis had decided to order a gallbladder ultrasound because she wasn't recovering as expected, and the ultrasound showed gallstones. Ms. Bevins reminded me of the "three Fs" mnemonic I had learned for COMLEX Level 1: fat females in their forties were prone to developing gallstones.

I wasn't scrubbed, gowned, and gloved. I stood outside the sterile field to observe the procedure on the video monitor. Ms. Bevins was unconscious, lying supine on the operating table. She had instruments and the laparoscope inserted into four abdominal ports. Her abdomen was insufflated (filled with gas) to expand the cavity for operation. Dr. Davis was assisted by a female scrub tech, who controlled the laparoscope and one of the instruments. Country music was playing.

"What's the triangle of Calot?" Dr. Davis asked me as he was blunt dissecting with a grasper.

"The area between the inferior margin of the liver superiorly, the cystic duct laterally, and the common hepatic duct medially," I said.

"Okay. What's this?" He touched the anatomy with a grasper.

"The cystic artery."

"Are you sure you want to go into psychiatry? You know your anatomy well."

"I enjoyed anatomy, and I briefly considered orthopedic surgery, but I figured I'd be miserable in residency and never see my wife."

"My wife didn't seem to mind not seeing me much during residency."

"That doesn't surprise me," the scrub tech said.

"Did I ask for comments from the peanut gallery?" Dr. Davis said. "Residency did suck. I worked hundred-hour weeks, but I pushed through 'cause I love surgery."

He placed a clip on the cystic duct to prevent stones from going into the common bile duct. He injected dye contrast into the cystic duct below the clip for a cholangiogram (x-ray of the bile ducts), which showed no stones in the common bile duct.

He placed two more clips on the cystic duct and cut the duct with scissors below the top clip, then followed the same procedure for the cystic artery. He used electrocautery to remove the gallbladder from the bottom of the liver, placed the gallbladder in a bag, and pulled it through a large port.

I left the room, rounded on patients on the surgical floor, and met Dr. Davis in the doctors' room. As I was updating him on the patients, my phone vibrated. Lynn was calling.

"Hello," I said.

"James, I just started bleeding!" she said frantically. "What should I do!"

"I'm sorry. Are you at work?"

"Yes."

"Call Dr. Border's office and ask if she can see you right away."

"Okay. I love you."

"I love you too. Bye."

She called me back after a few minutes. "I'm on my way to Dr. Border's office right now."

"Okay. I'll meet you there."

"That was my wife," I told Dr. Davis. "She's seven weeks pregnant. She just started bleeding, and she's on her way to her ob-gyn's office."

"I'm sorry," he said. "Get out of here. Go be with your wife."

"Okay."

I rushed to Dr. Border's office and met Lynn in an exam room. She was wearing a gown, sitting on an exam table with a disposable absorbable pad under her. The pad was soaked with blood.

"The bleeding won't stop!" she said, scared, crying.

"I'm sorry, babe." I held her hand.

Dr. Border entered the room. She appeared middle-aged, with long, brown hair streaked with dark magenta. She was wearing green scrubs, several earrings in each ear, a nose piercing, and she had tattoos on her arms and forearms.

"How are you doing?" she said to Lynn.

"Not good!" Lynn said. "The bleeding just started about 20 minutes ago, and it won't stop!"

"I'm sorry." Dr. Border said. She turned to me. "Can you take her to the hospital?"

"Of course," I said.

"I need to go to the hospital!" Lynn said.

"Yes. I'll meet you there," Dr. Border said.

"She needs surgery," I said.

"Yes."

We left the clinic, and I rushed her to BMC. I knew Lynn needed surgery because she was bleeding from an ectopic (tubal) pregnancy. The ultrasound that had been done the week before didn't show an embryo in the uterus. If the embryo had been seen in a fallopian tube, Lynn could have been treated with methotrexate.

We checked in at the ED, and we were quickly taken to a bed.

"I'm scared," Lynn said.

"I know." I held her hand.

"I wanted this so bad! I'm sorry!" She was crying again.

"It's not your fault."

"I feel like it is."

"It's not."

"Ow!"

A nurse kept poking her to try to start an IV line. Thankfully, she finally gave up, and an anesthesiologist came and quickly started the line. A bag of fluid was connected to the line with a fast drip, and IV Versed was given.

"What did they just give me?" she said. "I'm feeling much better now."

"Versed. It's good stuff."

A nurse came to the bed. "We're going to take you back now."

"Okay," Lynn said. "I love you, James."

"I love you too." I kissed her.

The nurse started rolling her bed away.

"Let me tell you about all my husband's secrets," Lynn said to the nurse with mildly slurred speech.

I smiled and went to a waiting room. My classmate David Blankenship and his wife, Rachel, Lynn's friend, sat with me for a while, and I thanked them for being supportive. Waiting was hard, of course, and it seemed like I had to wait for a long time. I was finally told Lynn was out of surgery, and I went to her room on the seventh floor. The window blind was mostly closed, and the room was dark. Only a light over the head of her bed was on. She was lying in bed, wearing a hospital gown.

"Hi, babe. How are you feeling?" I said.

"She had to cut me open." She showed me a bandage across her lower abdomen. She had a left salpingectomy (removal of the fallopian tube).

"I'm sorry."

"It really hurts." She pressed a button to receive an IV morphine dose from a pump. "I guess it's too early for another dose."

"I'm sorry."

"I'm so sad." She cried.

"I'm sad too." I sat on the side of the bed, held her hand, kissed her, and I cried too.

"I love you so much, James."

"I love you too."

Lynn was discharged the next day, and I took her home.

I observed another lap chole, and I was allowed to assist with a loop colostomy[19] for an 86-year-old male with rectal and lung cancer. The procedure was done for palliative care to divert stool from the rectum, which was obstructed by cancer. Dr. Davis made a midline incision from just beneath the breastbone to just above the pubic bone and dissected through deeper layers of fascia. I held retractors while he performed the surgery, which didn't take long. It was impressive to see an open abdomen for the first time: the yellow, fatty greater omentum hanging over the pink intestines like an apron; the colon extending up the right side, across the upper abdomen, then down toward the rectum; and the small intestine, which is about 20 feet long. As Dr. Davis was closing the incisions, he allowed me to do some suturing, but he quickly took back over because I wasn't quick enough, even though I had practiced with surgical towels.

The next day I observed scopes and rounded on patients. One of the patients was an alcoholic 70-year-old male with hematemesis (vomiting of blood), hematochezia (bloody stools), and cirrhosis (damaged, scarred liver). His EGD showed esophageal varices (dilated veins) and gastritis. The varices were caused by portal hypertension, which was caused by the cirrhosis, and they were prone to ulceration and massive bleeding. I couldn't believe the man had lived so long with such severe alcoholism. He certainly didn't have much time left. A 55-year-old alcoholic male was also admitted to the surgical floor with hematemesis. I wondered if he would live to age 70.

Lynn stayed home for the rest of the week to recover from surgery. She had significant pain, which worsened with movement. The older minister from a small Church of Christ we attended became aware of her ectopic pregnancy. We thanked him for praying for us, and we asked him to keep the news private. On Sunday morning, however, he violated our trust by sharing the news with the congregation, so we decided not to return. Lynn was raised as a Catholic, and we didn't like the church anyway. On another Sunday morning, when the minister was closing the worship service, he encouraged members to return for the evening worship service by saying, "Come back tonight to hear about the sin that leads unto death."

I only observed a few more surgeries during the rest of November: two lap choles and a loop ileostomy (small bowel opening in the abdominal wall) for a 34-year-old male, who had a partial colectomy (colon removal) for colon cancer. On weekdays I continued to round on patients on the surgical floor.

The air turned colder, the leaves fell to the ground, the mountains turned gray, and the days quickly became dark. I felt SAD (seasonal affective disorder) creep in. I wanted to sleep longer, and I felt loss of motivation, interest, and energy. Late autumn and winter in Brighton were depressing to me. I didn't feel this way when I lived in Hansen, Tennessee. The city wasn't closed in by gray mountains, so it didn't get dark as soon, and I liked the open landscape better—rolling hills with mountains in the distance.

At the beginning of December, I assisted with a colostomy takedown (colostomy reversal) for Tammy Compton, a 39-year-old female.

"It looks like a bomb went off in here!" Dr. Davis said after he opened her abdomen with a midline incision.

Her abdomen had many adhesions (inflammatory bands of scar tissue) from prior surgeries. Adhesions occur in at least 66% of patients who have had abdominal surgery and 90% of patients who have had two or more surgeries. Adhesions are the most common cause of small bowel obstruction in Western industrialized nations. Dr. Davis tediously manipulated the small intestine inch by inch with his fingers to tease apart the adhesions.

My low back started to hurt, and my arms started to fatigue and tremble from holding retractors for so long. I could hike for miles without back problems, but standing for long periods really hurt my back, and my lumbar spine would crunch and crackle when I bent forward to try to relieve the pain. This surgery was taking much longer than any other surgery I had observed. After Dr. Davis finally finished with the adhesions, he reconnected the colon by anastomosis (surgical union) and closed the abdomen. The surgery took about three hours, and I was glad when it was over.

The next day I observed scopes and rounded on patients. When I reviewed Ms. Compton's chart, I noticed that she also had a diagnosis of bipolar 1 disorder, and her medications included Risperdal (antipsychotic) and lithium (mood stabilizer). I knocked on her door.

"Come in," she said.

I opened the door, entered the dim room, and used hand sanitizer from a wall dispenser. Ms. Compton was reclined in bed with the head tilted up. She appeared older than her stated age, ill, disheveled, with red hair, wearing a hospital gown.

"Good morning, Ms. Compton," I said. "How are you feeling?"

"How do you think I'm feeling?" she said.

"Well, you just had a major surgery, and you had a lot of scar tissue in your abdomen from prior surgeries, so you're probably feeling pretty bad."

"I feel like fucking shit!"

"I'm sorry."

"Is Dr. Davis going to see me today?"

"Yes. Could I take a look at your incision?"

"Go ahead." She pulled up her gown.

I carefully lifted one side of her bandage, examined her incision without touching it, and gently pressed the bandage back into place.

"The incision looks good," I said. "Thank you. Dr. Davis should see you soon."

"Okay."

Later I returned with Dr. Davis to see her, but he stopped me outside the door to her room.

"I'll see Tammy," he said. "She doesn't want to see you again."

"I'm sorry," I said. "What did I do?"

"You didn't use gloves when you examined her."

"That's true, but I used hand sanitizer, and I didn't touch the incision. I'm sorry I upset her."

"It's okay. She's bipolar, and she can be difficult to deal with."

I felt really bad about pissing off Tammy Compton, and I did my best not to piss off other patients for the rest of December. I continued to observe scopes, lap choles, other surgeries, and I rounded on patients. The temperature started to dip into the 30s and below freezing. Lynn and I started attending a Methodist church in downtown Brighton. We enjoyed a Bible class led by a BCSOM pharmacology professor who had a gift for teaching, and some other medical students were in the class. I was thankful that Dr. Davis told me to take Christmas Eve and Day off. We enjoyed a visit from Lynn's parents, who lived in North Carolina. They stayed at the Fairfield Inn because our small apartment's second bedroom was more like a closet. A cheap futon, metal desk, and small, particleboard bookcase were crammed into the room. During my first two years of medical school, I spent a lot of time in the room, studying.

I assisted with a right BKA (below knee amputation) for a 41-year-old disabled male who had infected hardware from prior surgery for a tibia fracture. Hardware had been replaced but became infected again, and he had been treated with multiple courses of antibiotics. He was so miserable and fed up with unsuccessful treatments that he just wanted his leg cut off.

He also quickly developed an opioid addiction after taking prescribed Lortab, followed by Percocet, then OxyContin. He overused, then abused OxyContin, progressing from crushing and snorting the medication to injecting it within six months. He purchased illicit OxyContin because he ran out of prescribed medication before refills were due. His pain management provider discontinued OxyContin after a second pill count was short, and his urine drug screen was positive for Xanax, which was not prescribed.

This was another impressive surgery to observe. Dr. Davis cut through skin, fascia, and calf muscle above the hardware.

He used electrocautery to stop bleeding, and he ligated larger vessels. The smell of burning flesh was stronger, compared to other surgeries. When he got down to the tibia and fibula, he used an electric saw to finish the job. The amputation was also bloodier than other surgeries. Seeing the bloody stump and severed leg was kind of surreal, like a scene out of a horror or war movie. Dr. Davis placed the leg in a red biohazard waste bag, and he bandaged the stump without closing the incision. I felt sad for the man.

The incision was closed five days later. I was glad to complete my surgery rotation without pissing off another patient. Dr. Davis gave me a glowing evaluation, which surprised me, as I figured he'd just give me an okay evaluation. I thanked him for the experience. I would miss him too. I liked his sense of humor.

Endnotes

1. "Appy": appendectomy: surgical removal of the appendix.

2. Esophagogastroduodenoscopy (EGD): endoscopic examination of the esophagus, stomach, and duodenum (the first division of the small intestine).

3. Cholecystecomy: surgical removal of the gallbladder.

4. Stoma: an artificial opening in the abdominal wall that can be connected to the intestines or ureters via an ileal conduit (isolated segment of small intestine). The ureters are paired tubes that carry urine from the kidneys to the bladder.

5. A hepatobiliary iminodiacetic acid (HIDA) scan is a nuclear imaging procedure that is usually used to evaluate gallbladder function. It is also used to track the flow of bile from the liver to the small intestine.

6. A Mediport (or portacath) is a small medical appliance implanted beneath the skin. A catheter connects the port to a vein. The port has a septum through which drugs can be injected and blood samples can be drawn many times.

7. Biliary colic: intense pain usually felt in the right upper quadrant of the abdomen due to a gallstone blocking the cystic duct.

8. Hypokalemia: low potassium.

9. NPO: abbreviation for Latin phrase, meaning nothing by mouth.

10. Up to 40% of pancreatitis cases are caused by alcohol use.

11. One pint of Jack Daniels is equivalent to 10.67 servings of alcohol.

12. LFTs: liver function tests.

13. Versed (midazolam) is a sedative used for procedures.

14. Hypoxemia: deficient oxygenation of blood.

15. Hematoma: a mass of usually clotted blood that forms in a tissue, organ, or space as a result of a broken blood vessel.

16. Diverticulosis: presence of a number of diverticula (sacs) of the intestine, common in middle age.

17. Ileocecal valve: connection between the terminal ileum (small intestine) and colon.

18. Duodenum: first segment of the small intestine that extends from the stomach.

19. A loop colostomy is created by sewing a loop of colon to an opening in the abdominal wall and making a small hole in the loop to allow stool to exit into a colostomy bag.

Chapter 6

Obstetrics and Gynecology

I dreaded my ob-gyn rotation with Lindsey Border, M.D., in January. I was thankful Dr. Border saved Lynn's life, but it felt awkward to rotate with my wife's doctor. Lynn didn't like her bedside manner, streaked hair, piercings, and tattoos. I thought it would be cool to see some surgeries and "catch babies" being delivered, but I wasn't looking forward to examining female parts. I was averse to ob-gyn. Dr. Border was a graduate of the University of Kentucky's College of Medicine, and she had completed a grueling, four-year residency.

Dr. Border's clinic was a few miles from BMC. It was on the second floor of a three-story medical office building. I arrived at the front desk on Monday at 7:50 a.m. Dr. Border was standing in front of the desk, wearing a white lab coat and green scrubs, and she was looking at paperwork. A nurse was behind the desk.

"Good morning," I said.

"Hey," Dr. Border said. She looked back down at her paperwork, and she appeared to care less whether I was there. "How was your weekend?" she said to the nurse.

"It was good, but it went by too fast as usual," the nurse said. "How was your weekend?"

"I was on call."

"Sorry."

"Yeah. I'm tired, and I need a break from medical students. I wish I could cancel clinic and go home."

"Well, thanks for letting me rotate with you," I said.

"Uh-huh," Dr. Border said. She gave the paperwork to the nurse, and I followed her to an exam room.

We only spent about two minutes with the first 62-year-old patient. She had a positive HPV (human papillomavirus) DNA test, which indicated a high risk of developing cervical cancer, but her Pap smear was normal. HPV is the most common sexually transmitted infection in the U.S. We spent a few more minutes with Amber Taylor, the second 26-year-old patient. She was sitting in a chair, and she appeared attractive, well-groomed and well-dressed, with long, brown hair. Dr. Border didn't introduce me to the patients, so, of course, I felt more awkward.

"How are you?" Dr. Border said to Amber.

"I'm okay," Amber said. "Just a little nervous about how my Pap smear turned out."

"I know. Well, your test showed moderate cervical dysplasia."

"What does that mean?"

"We need to schedule you for surgery."

"Really! I've never had surgery before! Do I have cancer!" She appeared frightened.

"No, but moderate dysplasia has a high risk for turning into cervical cancer, so it should be removed."

"How would you remove it?"

"You need a LEEP.[1] It's a minor procedure."

"Okay. Could you tell me more about it?"

"I'll give you a local anesthetic and use a small electrical wire loop to remove the bad tissue. You'll be able to go home after the procedure."

"Okay. That doesn't sound so bad."

"It's not. Any other questions?"

"No."

"Okay. We'll get you scheduled."

We left the room and saw two patients for obstetric exams and one patient for a Pap smear.

We stopped outside an exam room door.

"This patient just sees me," Dr. Border said. "You can go ahead and see the next one. Just don't see patients with red flags and don't do breast or pelvic exams."

"Of course," I said. I went to see the next patient who had a green flag pulled next to her door. She was a 31-year-old OB (obstetric) patient. I entered the room. She was sitting on the exam table, and she appeared older than her stated age, obese, casually dressed.

"Ms. May. Hello," I said. "I'm James. I'm a medical student."

"Hi. Nice to meet you," she said.

"How are you?"

"I'm making it."

"Could you lie back and lift up your shirt?"

"Yeah." She lied down and lifted up her shirt to expose her abdomen.

I auscultated the fetal heart and measured the fundal height from the pubic symphysis to the top of the uterine fundus, but I wasn't confident with my measurement of 29 centimeters. Palpation was difficult due to her obesity. The fundal height exam is used from 16–18 weeks of gestation until 36 weeks of gestation to measure the growth of the fetus. Fundal height roughly corresponds to gestational age. The patient was at 26 weeks gestation, so her fundal height should have been 26 cm. Deviation of more than 2 cm (less than 1 inch) in fundal height measurement from that expected at a particular gestational age should prompt repeat measurement and may lead to further evaluation. A deviation of 4 cm or more is of great concern and requires further evaluation, including ultrasound assessment. I observed Dr. Border do two fundal height exams, but she offered me no instruction.

"Okay," I said. "Dr. Border will be in shortly."

"Okay. Thanks." She pulled her shirt down.

I left the room and saw a 23-year-old OB patient, then a 44-year-old GYN (gynecologic) patient with Dr. Border.

The GYN patient had vaginal discharge after endometrial ablation for menorrhagia (profuse menses). Dr. Border did a quick exam and reassured her that her discharge was normal.

I returned to see the 31-year-old OB patient with Dr. Border.

"How are you?" Dr. Border said to her.

"I've been better," she said. "We're going to have to put this baby up for adoption. I told Johnny we can't have another kid. We've already got five, and there's no way we can take care of another one."

"Well, that's a big decision. What does Johnny think about it?"

"He wants to keep the kid, of course, but we can barely keep food on the table and pay the bills. We've had our electricity cut off more than once. And I just can't handle another kid. I'm the one who has to deal with them most of the time. Johnny just plays video games and hangs out with his friends."

"Sounds like Johnny needs to get off his ass."

"You've got that right! I've told him to get a job 'cause our disability checks aren't enough, and he spends too much money on beer."

"Could you recheck her fundal height?" I said to Dr. Border. "I'm not sure if my measurement is right."

"Did they not teach you how to do this in medical school?" Dr. Border said.

"I know how to do the exam, but the measurement can vary by a few centimeters, depending on where exactly you place the tape measure at the pubic symphysis and where you palpate the top of the uterine fundus."

She rolled her eyes and rechecked the fundal height. She crossed through my "29 cm" measurement in the paper chart and wrote "26 cm." We left the room and saw the 23-year-old OB patient. Dr. Border rechecked her fundal height and corrected the measurement in her chart.

"Could I hear my baby's heart?" the patient said.

"Sure," Dr. Border said. She placed gel on the abdomen and used a handheld Doppler ultrasound device to auscultate the heart. Rapid thumping and whooshing came through the device's speaker.

"I love that sound!" The patient smiled brightly. "My little baby's heart."

I saw 19 patients on my first day in the clinic, including a pregnant 17-year-old and a 30-year-old who had a colposcopy (stereomicroscopic exam of cervix, vagina, and vulva) due to having a Pap smear that showed ASCUS (atypical squamous cells of undetermined significance). I was glad when my first day was over.

The next day I met Dr. Border at BMC to observe surgeries. The first case was a C-section for a 26-year-old. I was scrubbed, gowned, and gloved for the procedure, but I wasn't allowed to assist. The patient was lying on the operating table, conscious. She had been given spinal anesthesia, and a drape was between her head and abdomen. Dr. Border made a lower abdominal transverse incision and used electrocautery to stop bleeding. A female scrub tech assisted her, dabbing blood with a sterile white towel, passing instruments, and holding retractors.

"What's that smell?" the patient said as she detected her burning flesh.

"I'm just stopping the bleeding from your incision," Dr. Border said. "You're doing fine."

"Okay," the patient said.

Dr. Border dissected through deeper layers of fascia. Suddenly, she angrily slammed a metal instrument on the floor.

"Sorry," the scrub tech said. She had apparently passed her the wrong instrument.

Dr. Border grabbed a different instrument from the tray and didn't reply to her apology.

"Is everything okay?" the patient said.

"Yes, everything's going fine," Dr. Border said. She cut through the uterine wall, and amniotic fluid and blood were suctioned away.

"I feel pressure."

"Your girl's coming out now," Dr. Border pulled the baby out by the head.

"Already!"

"Yes."

The girl's nose and mouth were suctioned, the umbilical cord was clamped and cut, and the placenta was removed from the uterus. The girl was handed to another nurse, and she started to cry as the nurse cleaned her. She was then handed to her mother, who joyfully held her on her chest as her incisions were closed.

The C-section is the most commonly performed major surgery in the U.S., accounting for about 33% of all births. According to the American College of Obstetricians and Gynecologists (ACOG), the 60% increase in C-section rates from 1996 to 2011 "without clear evidence of concomitant decreases in maternal or neonatal morbidity or mortality raises significant concern that cesarean delivery is overused." Patient safety experts have said that too many pregnant women and their physicians in the U.S. schedule the surgery for convenience, and ACOG has recommended to safely reduce the primary (first) C-section rate. According to a study published in the Journal of the American Medical Association (JAMA) in 2015, the optimal rate should be 19%. According to the World Health Organization, the "ideal rate" should be 10–15%.

I assisted with two more surgeries on my second day: a left salpingo-oophorectomy (removal of the fallopian tube and its ovary) and tubal ligation. Later in the day I observed a vaginal delivery. The patient was an attractive, unmarried, 19-year-old primigravida (woman pregnant for the first time). She was in a delivery room on a bed with her feet in stirrups, and she had been given epidural anesthesia. Her face and hair were wet with sweat, and she was wearing a hospital gown. A nurse was holding her hand, and Dr. Border was sitting on a rolling stool between her legs.

"You're doing good," the nurse said.

"Give another push," Dr. Border said.

She yelled as she gave another push, and the baby's head crowned (distended the vaginal opening). "The epidural's not working worth a shit! I can feel the pain!"

"I'm sorry. Relax," Dr. Border said. "Breathe."

She breathed heavily.

"Okay. Push."

She growled and pushed again. The head advanced a little, and she defecated.

"Relax. Breathe."

She breathed heavily.

"I never should have let that motherfucker fuck me!" she said angrily. "He said we'd be together forever, but he just wanted to get his dick wet. I'll take his sorry ass to court for child support."

"You've got to do what you've got to do. Push."

She growled and pushed. The head advanced more, and she defecated again.

"Okay. Breathe."

She breathed heavily.

"We're almost there. Give another push."

"I can't." She appeared exhausted, and she cried.

"Yes you can. Think about how angry you are with that motherfucker and push!"

She screamed with rage and pushed harder.

"Okay. One more time."

She growled and pushed.

Dr. Border grabbed the baby by the head and pulled.

"Okay. Your boy is out."

"Thank God!"

Dr. Border suctioned the boy's nose and mouth and handed him to the nurse. Dr. Border clamped and cut the umbilical cord and removed the placenta from the uterus. The nurse cleaned the boy, he started crying, and he was handed to his mother.

"He's beautiful!" she said, crying.

The next day I saw 21 patients in the clinic. I was allowed to do a breast exam and Pap smear on a 71-year-old patient who was having an annual GYN exam. I palpated her breasts with circular motion, and I didn't feel any masses.

Another GYN patient was a very attractive, 30-year-old pharmaceutical sales representative who was scheduled for a Pap smear. She was sitting in a chair in an exam room. She had long, brown hair, and she was well-groomed and well-dressed, wearing heavy makeup, a fashionable black suit, and white blouse, which was stretched by large breasts.

"How's it going?" Dr. Border said.

"Okay. How are you?" she said.

"Tired, but I'm making it. Did you have a boob job?"

"Yes. This takes some getting used to. Could you take a look at them to see what you think?"

"Is it okay if he's in here?"

"That's fine."

"Okay. Hop up here."

She sat on the exam table. As she removed her jacket and blouse, I noticed she was wearing a wedding ring, and I wondered why she had breast augmentation. Did she want to please her husband? Was she insecure? Or did she hope that larger breasts would influence more male doctors to prescribe her company's medication? Maybe she had the surgery for all three reasons. She removed her bra, and Dr. Border palpated her breasts and examined the scars along the breast creases under the breasts.

"They look good to me," Dr. Border said. "What does your husband think?"

"He's happy," she said.

"Well, good."

"What do you think?" the patient asked me.

"I'd say your surgeon did a good job." I smiled.

"Thanks." She smiled and put her bra and blouse back on.

"Okay," Dr. Border said. "Now I need to look at you down there."

She removed her pants and underwear, and Dr. Border did her Pap smear.

On Thursday I continued the clinic grind, and I observed another vaginal delivery for a 22-year-old who required an episiotomy, an incision of the perineum to enlarge the vaginal opening.

I was glad when Friday arrived, and I was glad there was no clinic on Fridays. I assisted with two laparoscopic tubal ligations, and I observed a LEEP for the 26-year-old with moderate cervical dysplasia, and a total abdominal hysterectomy and bilateral salpingo-oophorectomy (TAH-BSO) for a 52-year-old with cervical carcinoma in situ (precancerous epithelial lesion). I happily returned home early to enjoy a weekend break from ob-gyn. Lynn returned from work shortly after 5 p.m., and she awakened me from a nap on the couch.

"I'm sorry," she said. "Did I disturb another nap?"

"I just had surgeries today. No clinic," I said.

"I wish I could leave work early."

"I'm counting down till this rotation is over."

"So you don't care for Dr. Border either?" She sat on the couch.

"No. On the first day she said she needed a break from medical students. She acts like she could care less whether I'm with her. She doesn't do any teaching. She's moody, childish, and she throws tantrums in the OR. I heard she even got into trouble once for actually hitting a nurse."

"Wow."

"Yeah. She makes the other doctors I've rotated with look awesome."

"Sorry, babe."

"Me too. Seeing deliveries, surgeries, and fake breasts is definitely interesting, but—"

"Fake breasts?"

"A drug rep had a boob job, and Dr. Border examined her breasts."

"A drug rep, huh? I bet she was pretty. Did you examine her tits too?"

"I didn't touch them."

"Good."

"She asked my opinion though."

"Seriously!"

"Yeah."

"And what did you say?"

"I said her surgeon did a good job." I smiled.

"Seriously!"

"Yes."

"So she was pretty. Did her fake tits turn you on?"

"I thought they were too big. I like your real tits."

"You better!" She slapped my arm.

"Come on. She's married, and I'm not going to have an affair with a patient."

"Being married doesn't necessarily mean anything. Maybe she'd rather have a doctor husband. Lots of women want to marry doctors. If some drug rep tries to take my man, I will kill the bitch!"

"Okay, babe."

"I'm serious."

"I know."

"I would be homicidal."

"I'm sure you would." I thought Lynn was cute when she acted jealous. "Anyway, the other thing I was going to say is that clinic is also drudgery. I'm just repeatedly doing OB exams and observing GYN exams."

"So the drug rep must have been a nice break from the drudgery."

"Yeah. She was really sexy, and I want to run away with her."

"Go ahead. I'll take half of all your future earnings."

"Seriously, I'm still not sure about my fundal height measurements, and Dr. Border is no help, of course. Do you think I want to do OB exams after what you just went through?"

"I'm sorry. It's my fault."

"It's not your fault."

"I've just always wanted to be a mom since I was a little girl." She became tearful.

"I know this has been really hard for you, but it's hard for me too. I've been sad too."

"I'm sorry. I love you."

"I love you too." I hugged her. Our cheeks touched, and I felt her tears.

I enjoyed a relaxing weekend with Lynn. A few inches of snow accumulated on the ground on Saturday. I felt less SAD when the gray mountains turned white. They were beautiful again for a short while. On Sunday at dusk, we saw an ambulance with flashing lights at an adjacent apartment building. A neighbor from our building told us the ambulance was there for his aunt who died of an overdose.

I continued to examine pregnant abdomens and watch GYN exams, which had no educational benefit, but I didn't mind because I had no interest in doing pelvic exams. I got a taste of assembly-line medicine one day in the clinic when I saw 42 patients, including a pregnant 14-year-old! I assisted with a lap tubal, hysteroscopy, and D&C (dilation of the cervix and curettage, a scraping of the uterine lining). I observed another C-section, then I was allowed to assist with a C-section. Dr. Border did some vaginal deliveries without me, so I asked labor and delivery nurses to call me if she had more deliveries.

I observed a TAH-BSO for a 43-year-old who had a left ovarian cystic teratoma, abdominal pain, and abnormal uterine bleeding. A cystic teratoma is a tumor that is usually benign but creepy. It contains well-differentiated tissues from the three embryonic germ cell layers (ectoderm, mesoderm, endoderm). The patient's tumor was about the size of a golf ball, and it contained hair and teeth! Dr. Border did more vaginal deliveries without me, so I didn't bother to remind the labor and delivery nurses to call me for deliveries. I wouldn't get to catch babies, but I didn't mind.

One day in the clinic, I made the mistake of not measuring the fundal height of a 28-year-old OB patient who was at 32 weeks gestation. She was sitting on the exam table, and she appeared her stated age, well-groomed and well-dressed, with a protuberant abdomen. She was pleasant, talkative, a little anxious, and OCDish, and she had an ultrasound CD with her. The previous week she had paid cash to have an extra ultrasound done at another facility. The result was normal, so I wrote "32 cm" for the fundal height measurement in her chart, and I went to see other patients in the assembly line.

Dr. Border stopped me between patients as we were outside a row of exam rooms. She had a chart in her hand.

"The patient in room three said you didn't do an OB exam," she said.

"That's true," I said. "She had a normal ultrasound last week, so I noted a normal fundal height."

Dr. Border did not like my reply. Her face seethed with anger, and I felt a surge of fear, but at least she didn't punch me. She didn't say another word. She dramatically crossed through the "32 cm" I had written in the chart, and she wrote "33 cm." She then went to remeasure the fundal height of all the other OB patients I had seen, and she changed the numbers in all of their charts. I had made a *big* mistake! I felt like a terrible, dishonest idiot for not doing a fundal height exam on one patient— especially a high-maintenance patient. I had just made a bad rotation worse. At least I only had one week left.

I was surprised Dr. Border allowed me to assist with another C-section after I made her so angry. I persevered through my remaining days of the clinic grind. I was glad I didn't have another day with over 40 patients, but I continued to see 20–30 patients a day. I was delighted my rotation ended two days early due to Dr. Border going out of town! She didn't complete my evaluation on my last day. She told me to leave the form with a nurse. I thanked her for allowing me to rotate with her, and she went to see another patient. I hoped my evaluation wouldn't be too bad, considering my false documentation, but I had a bad feeling about it.

As I left the clinic, I felt like jumping for joy for being done with Dr. Border! I wondered if she had chosen the wrong medical specialty, as she usually appeared miserable. And if she needed a break from medical students and didn't care to teach, why was she still accepting students? Everything I learned on the rotation, I taught myself. Other medical students had good rotations with different ob-gyns and bad rotations with other doctors who were bad teachers. I happily went home and read about teratomas, intrauterine growth restriction, and fetal macrosomia (abnormally large body size) while Dr. Border was out of town.

Endnote

1. LEEP: loop electrosurgical excision procedure.

Chapter 7

Hospitalist Medicine

I was happy to start my hospitalist medicine rotation in February after a miserable January. I arrived at BMC on Monday at 6:20 a.m. while it was still very cold and dark outside, and I went to a small office on the third floor to meet the hospitalists during patient handoff. The office was so small, I wondered if it was previously a closet. Both doctors were wearing scrubs and white lab coats. Kenneth Akers, D.O., was standing, holding a cup of coffee and a patient list. Matas Lutkus, M.D., was sitting next to a desk with a computer, also holding a patient list. He had worked an overnight shift, and he was sharing patient information.

Dr. Akers was a graduate of BCSOM's third class in 2002, and he had completed a three-year internal medicine residency. He appeared young, overweight, unshaven. Dr. Lutkus appeared young and fit, clean-shaven. His blond hair was buzzed as short as a new military recruit, and he had a large scar on his scalp. He was a foreign medical graduate (FMG) with a medical degree from Lithuania, and he had completed an internal medicine residency in the U.S.

"Good morning," I said. "I'm James Banks. I'm supposed to start my rotation today."

"Good morning, James," Dr. Akers said. "So you're our next victim?" He smiled.

"I guess so."

"Hello. Nice to meet you," Dr. Lutkus said with an exotic accent.

"Nice to meet you," I said.

"What was your last rotation?" Dr. Akers said.

"Ob-gyn."

"I'm sorry. I hated ob-gyn."

"Me too. I'm glad it's over."

"What kind of doctor are you gonna be?"

"Psychiatrist."

"Really?"

"Yeah."

"Well, good. Dr. Lutkus could probably use your help. He's a little off."

"Isn't everyone a little off?" Dr. Lutkus smiled.

"I don't know. Are they?" Dr. Akers said. "That sounds like something a crazy person would say."

"Dr. Akers is a funny guy."

"Dr. Lutkus is a refugee from Soviet oppression."

"I'm from Lithuania, and I'm not a communist."

"You better not be 'cause you're in America now."

"God bless the U.S.A. Can I finish handoff now so I can go home?"

"Okay. Who's going to try to die on me today?"

"Hopefully, nobody. Ms. Salyers may act like she's going to die, but she'll probably just need more Ativan."

"Okay."

Dr. Lutkus discussed new admissions and overnight issues with other patients. He answered Dr. Akers's questions, and he left the room.

"I need some breakfast before I see anyone," Dr. Akers said. "You have morning report in a few minutes?"

"Unfortunately," I said.

"Okay. Well, Dr. Bailey has advised me not to hinder students from attending. You can meet up with me after you're done."

"Okay."

I went down to the medical library on the first floor, and I pretended to pay attention to a riveting lecture about COPD by Dr. Bailey. COPD was a common problem in Eastern Kentucky because so many people were addicted to cigarettes. I returned to the third floor and met Dr. Akers in the doctors' room, which was adjacent to the nurses' station. He was sitting in front of a computer, socializing with another doctor.

"How was morning report?" Dr. Akers said.

"It was a struggle to stay awake," I said. "Dr. Bailey's voice is so soft and soothing. He talked about COPD."

"That's a good topic. We see a lot of COPD exacerbations." His pager beeped, and he checked it. "You can see Mrs. Tackett and Ms. Hall."

"Just two patients?"

"That should be plenty to get you started."

"Okay."

He picked up a phone to make a call.

I felt overwhelmed when I reviewed Mrs. Tackett's chart. She was 42 years old, and she had been transferred from Huntington Medical Center (HMC) in West Virginia on January 31 for debility (weakness). She was initially admitted to AVMC—where I had worked with Dr. Coleman—on January 8 for a laparoscopic ovarian cystectomy (cyst removal). She also had adhesions removed during the procedure, and she was discharged the same day. After discharge she quickly developed abdominal pain, nausea, and vomiting.

She was readmitted to AVMC, diagnosed with a bowel perforation and peritonitis (inflammation of the peritoneum, the membrane that lines the abdominal cavity), and she had a sigmoidectomy (removal of the sigmoid colon) with colostomy. She then developed acute respiratory failure and septic shock. She was intubated, and she received hemodialysis for acute renal failure. She was on multiple antibiotics, and she was started on Xigris for septic shock, but the medication was stopped after a head CT showed a left frontal lobe hemorrhage.

She stayed in AVMC for 10 days, then she was transferred to HMC for 11 days for more intensive care and a neurosurgery evaluation. The neurosurgeon determined that the hematoma was too small to cause significant problems, and surgery was not recommended. She was extubated on January 21, re-intubated on January 22, then successfully re-extubated on January 25. She was transferred from the ICU to a medical floor for two days. Antibiotics were tapered, then she was transferred to BMC on Levaquin and Flagyl. The discharge summary recommended to discontinue antibiotics on February 4. Cultures from JP surgical site drainage were negative. Serial blood cultures were also negative from January 23–27. Sputum culture showed Candida albicans, and she was given nystatin for thrush. She was also diagnosed with anemia and thrombocytopenia (low platelets).

Xigris was FDA-approved for adult patients with severe sepsis (sepsis associated with acute organ dysfunction) who were at high risk of death (APACHE II score ≥25). The medication was a recombinant form of activated protein C that had anti-inflammatory, pro-fibrinolytic (clot busting), and anti-thrombotic (anti-clot) properties. Eli Lilly and Company aggressively marketed Xigris, but there was weak evidence to support its use, and on October 25, 2011, the company withdrew the medication from the worldwide market after a major clinical trial failed to show a survival benefit for patients with severe sepsis and septic shock.

I was relieved that Ms. Hall, a 66-year-old female, only had shortness of breath, following a canthoplasty (aesthetic procedure to tighten the lower eyelids). She had COPD and a 100 pack-year smoking history (2 packs per day for 50 years).

I went to see Mrs. Tackett. She was asleep in bed, and she had a central line in her left subclavian vein connected to a bag of lactated Ringer solution (balanced crystalloids) for hydration and smaller bags of Levaquin and Flagyl. She had a dialysis catheter in her right jugular vein. She appeared her stated age, thin, pale, with messy, sandy blonde hair. Her husband was sitting in a chair, watching TV with the volume low.

"Hello," I said. "I'm James. I'm a medical student working with Dr. Akers."

"Good morning, James," he said.

"What's your relation?" I had learned to never assume how people were related to patients.

"I'm her husband."

"Okay."

He touched Mrs. Tackett's shoulder. "Honey, a medical student is here to see you."

She awakened.

"Mrs. Tackett. Good morning," I said. "I'm James. I'm a medical student working with Dr. Akers."

"Hi. What time is it?" she said.

"Almost nine o'clock."

"Thanks. I don't even know what day it is anymore. One day runs into the next."

"Well, you've been through a lot. It's amazing you're still alive."

"I guess. I've been through hell all because of a botched surgery, and I've been so sick, I wished I was dead."

"I'm sorry you've been through so much."

"Thanks. They told me I almost died in the ICU, and I had a near-death experience."

"Really?"

"Yeah."

"What was that like?"

"I was floating or flying outside of my body, like a spirit, moving toward bright, wonderful light. I felt completely at peace, and I had no pain."

"Sounds like that was quite an experience."

"It was."

"Do you believe in an afterlife?"

"Absolutely. I'm a Baptist."

"Okay. Well, how are you feeling?"

"Better than I was but still like I was run over by a Mack truck. My legs and arms are still really weak, and my right side is worse."

"Are you able to get to the bathroom?"

"No."

"Can you feed yourself?"

"No, but do you know when I'll be able to eat? I'm only allowed to have clear liquids."

"I'm not sure. I'll ask Dr. Akers, and he may want to check with the surgeon who did your colon surgery."

"Okay. Thanks."

"Sure. Could I take a look at your abdomen?"

"Yeah." She pulled covers down to her hips and pulled up her gown to expose her abdomen.

I used hand sanitizer from a wall dispenser, put on gloves, and examined her abdomen. She had a large, open wound with a JP drain in place and a colostomy bag. The wound appeared clean and non-erythematous (not infected). I auscultated her abdomen, heart, and lungs, and checked her motor (muscle) strength: 2/5 right, 3/5 left. She was able to move her right extremities but not against gravity, and her left extremities against gravity but not against resistance.

"Okay," I said. "Dr. Akers will see you soon."

"Okay. Thanks," she said.

I left the room and went to see Ms. Hall. She was sitting up in bed, watching TV, wearing oxygen by nasal cannula. She appeared older than her stated age, thin, heavily wrinkled, with dyed blonde hair, well-groomed and well-dressed. She had edema, erythema, and bruising around her eyes, and a few small sutures next to the lateral corners of her eyes.

"Ms. Hall. Good morning," I said. "I'm James. I'm a medical student working with Dr. Akers."

"Good morning," she said. "Aren't you a handsome, young doctor?"

"Thank you, but I'm not a doctor yet. How are you feeling?"

"Well, I'm not smothering anymore."

"That's good. You have COPD, and you're a smoker?"

"Yes, but I quit smoking."

"When did you quit?"

"When I came into the hospital." She smiled.

"Okay. Do you have oxygen at home?"

"Yes, but I haven't been using it like I'm supposed to. I hope I can go home today. I can't smoke in here, and this patch isn't cutting it. I'm dying for a cigarette."

"Okay. Let me take a listen to you." I auscultated her heart and lungs. Her lungs had decreased breath sounds due to COPD. "I'll tell Dr. Akers you want to go home today."

"Okay. Thank you."

"You're welcome."

I left the room and went to meet Dr. Akers. He wasn't in the doctors' room, but Dr. Davis was in the adjacent nurses' station, chatting with a nurse.

"Hi, Dr. Davis," I said.

"What's happening?" he said.

"I'm on a hospitalist rotation now."

"I'm sorry."

"It's okay so far. I just started today."

"Well, I'd probably need your psychiatric services if I had to manage diabetes and COPD exacerbations every day. I don't have the time anyway. I certainly appreciate our hospitalists helping with my patients."

"I just saw a patient who had a sigmoidectomy for a perforated bowel after she had a lap ovarian cystectomy, and she almost died from septic shock."

"That sucks."

"Yeah. Well, have a good day."

"Thanks. You too."

I went to the doctors' room and sat in front of a computer to spend more time reviewing Mrs. Tackett's chart as I waited for Dr. Akers. Daniel Keene, M.D., a family physician, entered the room and sat near me. He appeared older, balding, with dark hair, clean-shaven, wearing glasses, a red Oxford shirt, and brown pants. Dr. Keene was a talented musician. Lynn and I had seen him play banjo and sing with a bluegrass band during Brighton's annual Mountain Folks festival.

"What's the difference between love and herpes?" he said without introducing himself.

"I don't know," I said.

"Herpes lasts forever."

I laughed.

"What's green and eats nuts?"

"I don't know. A septic squirrel?"

"Gonorrhea."

I laughed. "I'm James."

"Nice to meet you, James. I'm Daniel."

"My wife and I saw you perform for Mountain Folks last year. You were good. We really enjoyed your band."

"Thanks. Jamming with the band is fun. It's good for a doctor to have a hobby. So you're a married man. What's the difference between a prostitute and a wife?"

"I don't know."

"A wife accepts credit cards."

I laughed and turned back to the computer. Dr. Akers entered the room after a while.

"Hi, Daniel," he said.

"Good morning," Dr. Keene said. "How are you today?"

"Okay. Just stamping out disease and saving lives. Have you told James any dirty jokes?"

"What do you think?"

"I think you can't help yourself."

"A doctor's got to have a sense of humor."

Dr. Akers sat next to me. "Okay. Are you ready to present Mrs. Tackett's case?"

I tensed up a little. Formally presenting cases to attending doctors was intimidating.

Dr. Akers's pager beeped, and he made a phone call. "Okay, give her 20 of potassium," he said.

I presented part of my summary of Mrs. Tackett's case.

Dr. Akers's pager interrupted me, and he made another phone call. "We have an admission."

"Okay."

"Go ahead and finish."

I finished my summary without another pager interruption.

"Okay. She had a GI[1] bleed, so what kind of anemia does she have?" he said.

"Iron-deficiency," I said.

"She had an acute GI bleed from a bowel perforation."

"So she wouldn't have iron deficiency. A chronic GI bleed from colon cancer or a peptic ulcer would cause iron deficiency."

"Okay. Is her anemia microcytic, normocytic, or macrocytic?"[2]

"Normocytic. Iron-deficiency anemia is microcytic."

"Okay. What are other causes of normocytic anemia?"

"Anemia of chronic disease, hemolytic anemia, aplastic anemia, chronic renal failure."

"What are other causes of microcytic anemia?"

"Thalassemia, sideroblastic anemia, lead poisoning."

"What causes macrocytic anemia?"

"B12 or folate deficiency."

"Okay. What can you tell me about sepsis?"

"Sepsis is diagnosed when a patient has an infection and systemic inflammatory response syndrome."

"What is SIRS?"

"Fever, tachycardia, tachypnea, and leukocytosis."[3]

"The patient could also be hypothermic or have leukopenia."

"Okay."

"What is severe sepsis?"

"Sepsis with organ failure."

"What is septic shock?"

"Sepsis with hypotension."

"Okay. Why did Xigris cause a cerebral hemorrhage?"

"I had to look that up. Xigris is activated protein C. It has anti-thrombotic and fibrinolytic properties, so it increases bleeding risk."

"How could those effects be beneficial with a particular complication of severe sepsis or septic shock?"

"They could reduce the risk clot formation from DIC,[4] but DIC can also cause bleeding."

"Exactly. Xigris is the only FDA-approved medication for severe sepsis, but it was narrowly approved, and it's a scary medication to use. Mrs. Tackett has a cerebral hematoma, but she's still alive, and she's fortunate to be able to walk and talk."

"For sure."

"How is Ms. Hall doing?"

"She's dying for a cigarette, and she's ready to go home."

Dr. Akers smiled, and we went to see the patients together. He ordered physical and occupational therapy for Mrs. Tackett, and he discharged Ms. Hall. We went to the ED to see the new admission, a 42-year-old male with right lower lobe pneumonia. Dr. Akers did a quick history and physical, and his pager beeped while he examined the patient. We returned to the third-floor doctors' room, and Dr. Akers made a phone call.

"She last had Ativan seven hours ago?" he said. "Okay. Give her another half milligram." He hung up the phone and turned to me. "This is the third time I've been paged for Ms. Salyers this morning. I spend 80 percent of my time on 20 percent of the patients."

"That's got to be frustrating," I said.

"It is what it is. Sometimes I feel like I need some Ativan."

I laughed.

"Flying is my Ativan."

"You're a pilot?"

"Yeah. I forget all about disease and death and all the pain-in-the ass patients when I'm up in the sky."

"Do you have your own plane?"

"Yeah. I have a V-tail Bonanza." He showed me an image of the plane on a computer.

"Cool."

"This plane has also been called the 'doctor killer.'"

"Well, that doesn't sound cool."

"It's faster than other single-engine planes."

"Okay. Do you fly often?"

"As often as I can. I'll be flying to Columbus this weekend to see my son."

"How long will that take?"

"About an hour and a half. The drive is five hours."

"Well, that will save a lot of driving time."

"Yes. My son lives with his mother. Medicine is a severe mistress."

"Medicine took a toll on your marriage?"

"My ex liked the idea of being married to a doctor, but she couldn't keep her vagina in her pants when I was working 80-hour weeks. I caught her with a guy who was young enough to be her son."

"Whoa."

"Yeah. I wasn't entirely surprised though. I was suspicious. I think she mostly just liked the money. We'll grab some lunch after I dictate this admission."

"Okay."

After Dr. Akers finished the dictation, we went to the cafeteria, and he bought my lunch. Medical students always appreciated free lunches. I thanked him, and we enjoyed a meal together. He didn't expect me to see any more patients. I was happy to have the rest of the day free, but I also felt a bit uncomfortable. I felt like I should see more than a few patients. In any case, the first day of my hospitalist rotation was *awesome* compared to the first day of my ob-gyn rotation!

On Tuesday Dr. Akers allowed me to see three patients, including Mrs. Tackett. I saw the 42-year-old male with pneumonia and a 47-year-old male with a foot ulcer due to poorly controlled DM, and they were both discharged. On Wednesday I started following two more patients: a 73-year-old female with CHF, atrial fibrillation (A-fib), OxyContin withdrawal, left BKA, and peripheral vascular disease (PVD) due poorly controlled DM; and a 90-year-old female with shortness of breath, acute exacerbation of COPD, and severe CHF. I couldn't believe the 90-year-old was still alive with a cardiac ejection fraction (EF) of 10%! EF is a measurement of the percentage of blood pumped out by the left ventricle, and normal EF is above 55%. On Thursday and Friday I continued to follow the three patients, and I saw a new patient each day.

When I started my second week, the three patients were no longer in the hospital. Mrs. Tackett had been discharged to a rehab facility, and the other patients had also been discharged. I started following a new patient who was much more interesting to me. Ms. Blair was 38 years old, and she had multiple sclerosis (MS) and schizoaffective disorder, a serious mental illness characterized by a blend of symptoms of schizophrenia and major depression or bipolar disorder. She was admitted for an MS exacerbation.

I knocked on her door.

"Come in," she said.

I entered the room. "Ms. Blair. Good morning. I'm James. I'm a medical student, working with Dr. Akers."

"Nice to meet you, James." She stumbled and nearly fell as she walked from the bathroom to her bed.

"Are you okay?"

"Yeah. I'm just really weak, and my legs are numb. I've got MS." She sat on the side of the bed. She appeared older than her stated age, disheveled, with blonde hair, wearing a hospital gown.

I used hand sanitizer from a wall dispenser, and I thought about Tammy Compton, the bipolar patient I pissed off during my surgery rotation. I was determined not to piss off Ms. Blair.

"Both legs are numb?" I said.

"Yeah," she said.

"And how about weakness?"

"Both legs."

"Have you had any balance difficulty?"

"Maybe. It's hard to tell when I feel like I can't control my legs."

"How about dizziness?"

"I'm always dizzy."

"When did your legs start feeling weak and numb?"

"After my boyfriend and I got into a fight."

"When was that?"

"Yesterday. I broke up with him. He was always drunk and talking down to me and treating me like crap."

"I'm sorry. How long were you together?"

"Two, maybe three months."

"Were you drinking too?"

"No. I can't drink on my meds."

"Okay. According to our records, you had your last brain MRI six months ago."

"That sounds about right."

"And Dr. Trivedi is your neurologist?"

"Yes. She's a good doctor."

"Good. Have you had any changes in vision?"

"No."

"Any problems with concentration or memory?"

"Nothing new. I always have difficulty staying focused and getting things done, and I'm always losing things."

"Okay. Do you mind if I examine you?"

"Sure."

I auscultated her heart and lungs and conducted a neurological exam. I asked her to follow my finger with her eyes to check extraocular movement, and I checked her pupil responses with a pen light. I asked her to squeeze my index and middle fingers to check her grip strength, and she flexed and extended her forearms against my resistance. I asked her to scoot back on the bed a little bit so that her feet weren't touching the floor, and she flexed and extended her legs against my resistance. I asked her to walk across the room and back. She walked slowly, and her legs buckled, but she caught herself and didn't fall.

I used a reflex hammer to check deep tendon reflexes in all her extremities. I tapped the brachioradialis tendons a few inches above the wrists. I placed my thumb on the biceps tendons and struck my thumb with the hammer, and I struck the triceps tendons directly. I checked her knee jerk, ankle jerk, and plantar reflexes. When I stroked the soles of her feet with the end of the reflex hammer handle to check her plantar reflexes, she jerked her legs and said, "That tickles!"

I checked sensation in all her extremities. She said she could feel light touch on her arms but not her legs, but she could distinguish between the dull and sharp end of a safety pin with light pricks. I checked vibratory sensation by placing a vibrating tuning fork on the balls of her great toes.

"Okay," I said. "Dr. Akers will see you in a little while."

"Okay. Thank you," she said.

I saw two more patients on Monday: Ms. Hatfield, an 82-year-old female with vascular dementia due to multiple strokes, urinary tract infection (UTI), dehydration, and dysphagia (difficulty swallowing); and Ms. McCoy, an 83-year-old female with an infected Mediport, bacteremia, and an ESBL Proteus mirabilis infection in her left eye. The bacteria produced extended spectrum beta-lactamase, an enzyme that destroys and inactivates most antibiotics.

I went to the doctors' room and presented the cases to Dr. Akers.

"What do you think about Ms. Blair?" he said.

"Well, she complained of weakness and numbness in both legs," I said. "I think it's unlikely an MS exacerbation would cause bilateral deficits, but she almost fell twice. Reflexes in upper and lower extremities were normal. She denied light touch sensation in her lower extremities, but she could distinguish between dull and sharp pricks, and vibratory sensation was intact. Also, I tickled her when I checked her plantar reflexes."

Dr. Akers laughed. "Okay. What's her diagnosis?"

"I'm not sure if she has an MS exacerbation. She said her symptoms started after she broke up with her boyfriend. Should she have another MRI? Her last one was done six months ago."

"That will be for Dr. Trivedi to decide. We'll order a consult." He smiled. "We know Ms. Blair well. She's having another pseudoexacerbation."

"Okay."

"She's a good case for medical students to see—especially you since you're going to be a shrink."

"She is interesting."

Dr. Trivedi saw Ms. Blair the following day. MS pseudoexacerbations last less than 24 hours, but Ms. Blair continued to complain of lower extremity weakness, numbness, and she demonstrated difficulty walking. She fell and landed on the side of her right thigh and butt for Dr. Trivedi, but she didn't hurt herself. Dr. Trivedi agreed that she was probably having another pseudoexacerbation, so she didn't need an MRI, and she would see her again the next day if she was still in the hospital. Dr. Akers decided to keep her in the hospital for another day. On Wednesday Ms. Blair said she was feeling much better. She walked without difficulty, and she was ready to go home, so she was discharged.

Ms. McCoy no longer had bacteremia, but she still had the nasty antibiotic-resistant Proteus eye infection. She was also diagnosed with protein malnutrition and dysphagia, and surgery was consulted for PEG tube placement. Ms. Hatfield had a PEG tube placed the day before due to dysphagia. A PEG tube allows nutrition to be delivered directly into the stomach through the abdominal wall. I also saw a 78-year-old female who developed a left lower extremity deep vein thrombosis (clot) after right hip open reduction internal fixation (ORIF) surgery for a fracture. She was discharged to a rehab facility.

On Thursday I saw five patients, and Ms. Hatfield was discharged. A 61-year-old female had an impressive number of diagnoses: anemia, CHF, DM, HTN, CAD with history of MI, CABG (coronary artery bypass graft) of five arteries, CKD (chronic kidney disease), PVD, neuropathy (nerve dysfunction due to damage), left Charcot foot, retinopathy (retina damage), right hemiparesis (partial paralysis) from a CVA (cerebrovascular accident, a stroke), and morbid obesity. She was a train wreck who illustrated the range of complications that develop as a result of poorly controlled DM and HTN. Charcot foot is a rare but serious complication caused by peripheral neuropathy, especially in patients with DM. Loss of proprioception (position sense) in the patient's foot gradually weakened the bones and joints of her foot and ankle, and her arch collapsed, causing a "rocker-bottom" deformity. She had a history of pressure ulcers over the deformity.

On Friday Ms. McCoy was discharged to a rehab facility.

On Monday I called Dr. Border's office because BCSOM hadn't received my evaluation from her. A nurse told me she would remind Dr. Border to complete the evaluation. I continued to stamp out disease and save lives over the next two weeks. I worked with another hospitalist, then Dr. Akers again for my last few days.

I saw a dying patient during my last two days. Mr. Daniels was a 41-year-old male with respiratory failure, a tracheostomy (surgical opening into the trachea through the neck), PEG tube, end-stage liver disease secondary to alcoholic cirrhosis, hepatic encephalopathy (delirium caused by nitrogenous wastes), and esophageal varices. He had been removed from a ventilator in the ICU and transferred to a room on the third (medical) floor. He was lying flat in bed, in a coma, and he appeared older than his stated age, thin, disheveled, unshaven, and jaundiced (yellowed skin caused by deposition of bile pigments). He was wearing oxygen by nasal cannula, and he had an IV bag connected to a bag of normal saline. He was receiving low-dose morphine every two hours to prevent him from becoming short of breath. He wasn't connected to a vitals monitor. I felt heavy when I was in the room, especially when Dr. Akers talked with his mother beside the bed.

"He has a fever, but I don't recommend starting an antibiotic," he said.

She started crying. "I told him the drinking was going to kill him if he didn't stop, but he just couldn't stay sober. I never stopped praying for him."

"I'm sorry," Dr. Akers said.

We stood in silence for a moment.

"We're keeping him comfortable," Dr. Akers said.

His mother touched his head and kissed his cheek. "I love you, son."

Dr. Akers and I left the room and went to see the next patient.

"Is it hard to just move on to the next patient after seeing a case like that?" I said.

"It never gets easy, but you have to get used to it," Dr. Akers said. "It's harder in the ICU. It's much more intense. Some patients aren't going to make it out of there, and some families are really difficult to deal with. They're very emotional, and they can't accept or understand a poor prognosis, so they want everything done. I'm happy to leave the critical care to the intensivists."

The patient was still breathing on my last day. At the end of the day, Dr. Akers gave me a good evaluation, and I thanked him for the experience, which was *far* better than ob-gyn.

Endnotes

1. GI: gastrointestinal.

2. The average size of red blood cells is smaller than normal with microcytic anemia, normal with normocytic anemia, and larger than normal with macrocytic anemia.

3. Tachypnea: abnormally rapid breathing. Leukocytosis: abnormally large number of white blood cells.

4. DIC: disseminated intravascular coagulation.

Chapter 8

Internal Medicine with Dr. Kazim

I started my internal medicine rotation with Ehsan Kazim, M.D., in March. His clinic was in Jonesboro, Kentucky, half an hour east of Brighton. The tiny town of 578 residents was separated from Jonesboro, West Virginia, by the Buffalo River. The West Virginia town had a population of 3,063. Dr. Kazim was an FMG with a medical degree from Pakistan, and he had completed an internal medicine residency in the U.S. He was in solo practice, and he rounded on his hospitalized patients, so he was on call 24-7. His wife was his office manager. The proportion of physicians in solo practice has declined from 18.4% in 2012 to 14% in 2020.

I arrived at the clinic front desk on Monday at 8 a.m., and a female receptionist took me to meet Dr. Kazim in the break room. He was standing in front of a wall-mounted TV, watching CNN coverage of Obama. He appeared middle-aged, overweight, handsome, with a well-trimmed beard. He was wearing a stethoscope around his neck, a lavender Oxford shirt, and gray pants.

"Dr. Kazim. Good morning," I said. "I'm James Banks."

"Good morning, James," he said with an exotic accent. "Welcome."

"Thank you."

"How are you?"

"Good. How are you?"

"Okay so far. We'll see how the day goes. Would you like some coffee and a pastry?"

"No thanks. I've already had my coffee for breakfast."

"You skip breakfast? It's the most important meal of the day."

"I'm not sure if there's any scientific basis for that claim."

"You're probably right, and that's probably why you're slim. Well, I'm going to have a delicious cinnamon roll and live it up for the rest of this week. I have to start fasting next week to lose this gut. My parents are coming to visit." He started eating a cinnamon roll and poured himself a cup of coffee. "You sure you don't want another cup of coffee?"

"I'm good. Thanks."

"Fasting is going to be *so* hard, especially with drug reps bringing lunch every day! I love food. What kind of medicine do you want to practice?"

"Psychiatry."

"Not many students go into psychiatry, but I think that's a good choice. Where do you want to do residency?"

"I'm not sure yet, but I plan to apply to university-based programs in Kentucky, Tennessee, North Carolina, and out West."

"Vanderbilt's in Tennessee."

"Yeah. I plan to apply there."

"That would be hard to get into Vanderbilt."

"I'm sure it is. I also plan to apply to Wake Forest, which is near my wife's parents."

"Wake Forest is also a great school. Why are you interested in western programs?"

"I lived in Colorado before. I love the West, and I'd like to live out there again."

"I haven't been to Colorado."

"The Rocky Mountains are awesome."

"I've seen pictures of Colorado. It does look awesome. Are you ready to see some patients?"

"Yeah."

"Okay. You can start with room one."

"Okay."

I left the break room and went to see the first patient, a 41-year-old obese female with an arthritis flare in her left knee. She appeared her stated age, well-groomed, casually dressed. I took a quick history, examined her knee, and left the room. I met Dr. Kazim and a young, tall, obese man in the hall. He appeared clean-shaven but otherwise disheveled. His brown hair was messy, and his clothes were wrinkled. He was wearing a white lab coat, khaki pants, and a light green polo shirt that was too small and not fully tucked in.

"You're late again," Dr. Kazim said to him.

"I'm sorry," he said. "I overslept."

"Maybe you need a sleep study."

"I probably do. I'm sorry. I'll do better."

"Kevin, this is James," Dr. Kazim said. "He's a medical student."

"Nice to meet you, Kevin," I said.

"Likewise," he said. "I'm an FNP[1] student."

"You can see the patient in two," Dr. Kazim said to Kevin.

"Okay," he said.

Dr. Kazim and I saw the patient with the arthritic knee. He carried a tablet computer with him, and he sat on a stool in front of the patient, who was sitting in a chair.

"How are you?" Dr. Kazim said.

"Okay, except for my knee," she said. "It's really been hurting. I've been limping around like an old lady."

"I'm sorry. You are in your 40s now."

"Do you have to tell me that?"

"Yes. I'm your doctor." He smiled. "You've also gained weight since your last appointment. You're supposed to be losing weight. You need to lose 60 pounds to get down to a normal weight."

"I know, but it's been too cold to get outside and walk."

"You can't put a coat on?"

"I don't like the cold."

"What's your diet like?"

"I don't eat that much."

"What kinds of foods do you eat?"

"I like McDonald's Big Macs and fries."

"Do you have Cokes with your Big Macs and fries?"

"Yes. The combo meal is a good deal."

"Coke is loaded with sugar. What else do you eat?"

"Meat and potatoes, fried chicken, spaghetti, pizza."

"What about fruits and vegetables?"

"Aren't potatoes vegetables?"

"Yes. What about other vegetables and fruit?"

"I don't care for fruit unless it's baked in a pie. I love pies. And I like fried vegetables, like okra, pickles, green tomatoes."

"Okay. Well, your diet sounds delicious, but it's full of high-calorie, high-fat foods, and sugar. You should have less McDonald's, fried foods, and pies, and more fresh fruits and vegetables. No more Cokes and no canned foods. Many canned foods are high in sodium and sugar. Your joints aren't designed to carry this much weight. If you don't lose weight, you could end up needing knee replacements, hip replacements, back surgery, and you'll probably have to start medications for diabetes and high blood pressure."

"Well, I sure don't want all of that. I'll try to do better."

"Good. You can take prescription strength ibuprofen as needed for pain and inflammation, and, hopefully, your knee will calm down soon. You can see me back in a month and call if you need to." He touched his tablet with a stylus to order the medication and complete the visit note.

"Okay. Thank you."

"You're welcome."

I noticed that Dr. Kazim didn't examine the patient's knee during the appointment. We went to see the next patient together, a 56-year-old obese female with HTN, left foot numbness, and history of back surgery in 2005. Her BP was well controlled, so Dr. Kazim saw her quickly, and we moved on to the next patient, a 67-year-old male with HTN.

"Your blood pressure's still high, unfortunately," Dr. Kazim said. "158 over 95, and you're on high doses of losartan, carvedilol, and hydrochlorothiazide." He turned to me. "James, can you tell me what classes these medications are in?"

"ARB,[2] beta blocker, and diuretic," I said.

"Okay. What other class of medication could we add?"

"Uh, a calcium channel blocker."

"Good job." Dr. Kazim smiled. "That's what sets you apart."

"What do you mean?"

"You answered correctly because you are a medical student. Kevin needs to study his pharmacology. Nurse practitioner and PA[3] students don't get as much education in pharmacology as medical students."

"Oh, okay."

Dr. Kazim prescribed amlodipine for the patient.

I thought the question was easy, compared to questions other doctors had asked me, but I was happy to impress Dr. Kazim. We saw a few more patients and had free lunch with Kevin at a long table in the break room. An attractive female drug rep provided pulled pork, barbecue chicken, slaw, baked beans, green beans, mashed potatoes, and apple cobbler. I loaded up my plate with pulled pork and all the sides. I was happy to be on another rotation with free lunches!

"I love pulled pork," I said.

"Me too," Kevin said.

"I can't eat pork," Dr. Kazim said. He was eating chicken.

"Why not?" I said.

"Swine are dirty animals," Dr. Kazim said.

"Are you Muslim?" I said.

"Yes."

"Okay."

Kevin and I enjoyed our swine, and, of course, we all enjoyed some apple cobbler for dessert. After the delicious, high-calorie, high-fat lunch, I felt like a slug in need of a nap. I called Dr. Border's office again because BCSOM still hadn't received my evaluation from her. A nurse told me she would again remind Dr. Border to complete the evaluation. I dragged myself to see more patients with DM, HTN, HLD, arthritis, upper respiratory infections, pneumonia, and I returned home.

The next day was busier as I started seeing hospitalized patients. Dr. Kazim rounded on patients at two hospitals in Jonesboro, Kentucky, and Jonesboro, West Virginia. Thankfully, I only had two patients to see at Jonesboro Medical Center (JMC) in Kentucky. I arrived at the hospital at 6:30 a.m., spent some time familiarizing myself with the EMR, then saw a 73-year-old female with dementia and pneumonia and a 90-year-old female with a right humerus fracture, fever, mild shortness of breath, and confusion. Dr. Kazim soon joined me, and we quickly saw the patients together. He ordered a chest x-ray and urinalysis for the 90-year-old, and he discharged the demented lady with pneumonia. The patients were easy, compared to the patients I saw in BMC!

We hurried back to the clinic, and Dr. Kazim stopped in the break room to grab a bite of breakfast and cup of coffee. Kevin was sitting at the table, eating a pastry.

"Good job, Kevin," Dr. Kazim said, smiling. "You're on time today."

"I told you I'd do better," Kevin said, smiling.

"I'm going to be good and have an apple this morning," Dr. Kazim said.

"I thought you were going to live it up this week," I said.

"I have to start eating better. No more cinnamon rolls, donuts, or apple cobbler. You guys have to keep me out of here next week. There's always bad food in here."

"I'll guard the entrance," Kevin said.

"I'm sure you will," Dr. Kazim said.

I left the room to see patients with GI, respiratory, cardiovascular, and musculoskeletal problems. One of the patients with nausea and vomiting, a 39-year-old female, had a kidney transplant. A 67-year-old female with HTN was on Coumadin due to a history of a portal vein thrombosis. (The portal vein is a large vessel that carries blood from the digestive tract and spleen to the liver.) Two of the patients with musculoskeletal problems had worked as coal miners. A 67-year-old male suffered from low back pain since a mining accident that occurred 17 years earlier. A 49-year-old male had arthritic pain in his hands and back and degenerative disc disease after working as a miner for 27 years.

During the morning I stopped in the business office between patients to catch Dr. Kazim, and his pretty, quiet wife handed me a small paperback book.

"This is for you," she said with an exotic accent.

"The Qur'an," I said. "I have the Bible, but I haven't read the Qur'an."

"It is an excellent book."

"I'll return it to you when I'm done with it."

"It is a gift."

"Oh, okay. Well, thank you."

"You're welcome."

The next day Kevin and I saw different hospitalized patients. I saw two new hospitalized patients at JMC: a 77-year-old female with abdominal pain and a partial diverticulosis perforation, and a 95-year-old female with a left ankle fracture and UTI. The 90-year-old lady with the humerus fracture had a chest x-ray and urinalysis, which showed signs of pneumonia and a UTI.

I drove across the Buffalo River to see one patient at Riverside Community Hospital (RCH) in West Virginia. RCH looked like a Section 8 facility, compared to JMC, which was a nice, newer facility. RCH was old, dingy, dimly lit, depressing, and only paper charts were used, which meant that I would probably have difficulty deciphering illegible doctors' notes. I reviewed the chart for Ms. Estep, and I was able to decipher that she was 84 years old, and she was admitted for syncope, digitalis toxicity, and renal failure. She was taking digoxin for CHF. Digoxin is a medication derived from the leaf of digitalis (common foxglove), a perennial flowering plant. Digoxin increases the force of heart contractions.

I entered Ms. Estep's room. She was sitting up in her hospital bed, and she grabbed at the air in front of her like she was trying to catch a bug. She appeared her stated age, with white hair, wearing a hospital gown and oxygen by nasal cannula. She had an IV line connected to a bag of normal saline and telemetry wires for cardiac monitoring.

"Ms. Estep. Good morning," I said. "I'm James. I'm a medical student working with Dr. Kazim."

"Good morning, James," she said.

"How are you?"

"I'm just lovely. How are you?" She smiled and grabbed at the air again. She looked unusually happy for someone who was suffering from digitalis toxicity.

"I'm okay, thanks. What's going on? What are you doing?"

"I'm catching lightning bugs. They're so beautiful. Do you have a jar to put them in?"

"I'm sorry. I don't. Can you tell me how you ended up in the hospital?"

"I can't be in a hospital. Lightning bugs aren't in hospitals."

"Well, I guess they're in this hospital. You're in Riverside Community Hospital. You were admitted after you fainted and fell, and your digoxin level is toxic."

"I don't remember falling, but I have felt dizzy."

"Do you remember if you may have taken too much of your digoxin?"

"I don't know. My daughter helps me with my medications because I get confused sometimes. You look kind of green like a lightning bug."

"Do I?"

"Yes. You have a glow about you. I'd like to put you in a jar. You're cute." She giggled.

I smiled. "Thanks. I don't think I'd fit in a jar. I need to examine you."

"Of course."

I palpated her radial pulse, auscultated her heart and lungs, examined her abdomen, and pressed on her legs to check for pitting edema.

"Are you married?" she said, smiling.

"Yes," I said.

"She must be a lucky woman."

"Or I'm a lucky man. Dr. Kazim will see you soon."

"Okay. Thank you." She smiled.

I left the room and went to a nurses' station computer to read an eMedicine article about digitalis toxicity while I waited for Dr Kazim. He soon arrived in a hurry.

"Good morning?" he said. "How is our patient?"

"She's delirious from the digitalis toxicity," I said. "She's catching lightning bugs, and she wants to put me in a jar."

"Really?" He laughed. "Why does she want to put you in a jar?"

"Because I'm cute, and I'm glowing like a lightning bug."

He laughed. "What's her digoxin level?"

"5.2."

"Okay. She had a syncopal episode prior to admission. How's her EKG?"

"It showed bradycardia with a rate of 45. Today her pulse is 52, and her blood pressure's okay."

"Okay. How are her labs?"

"Normal, except for creatinine of 3.5."[4]

"How's her physical exam?"

"Heart sounds are faint. Lungs are clear. Abdomen is soft and nontender. She has pitting edema in her legs."

"Okay. What are we going to do for her?"

"I was just reading about digitalis toxicity. I haven't yet seen a case of this. We should hold digoxin, continue IV hydration, monitor digoxin levels."

"Good job. What's the half-life[5] of digoxin?"

"One and a half to two days."

"Okay. Let's go see her."

We quickly saw Ms. Estep and rushed to JMC to see the other patients together. The 95-year-old lady with the left ankle fracture and UTI was discharged with an orthopedic boot and antibiotic. The 90-year-old lady with the humerus fracture was discharged with antibiotics for pneumonia and a UTI. The 77-year-old female with abdominal pain and partial diverticulosis perforation had an NPO order, and she was receiving IV antibiotics. We rushed to the clinic and saw more patients.

I continued to follow Ms. Estep and the 77-year-old for the rest of the week, and I had much busier clinic days (23 to 25 patients per day). On Thursday I saw patients in the Jonesboro clinic in the morning and in a rural West Virginia clinic in the afternoon. The rural clinic was half an hour away in the middle of nowhere, along a narrow, twisty mountain road. Dr. Kazim drove us there in his Mercedes sedan like Dr. Coleman—fast. We drove through Williamson, West Virginia, and I noticed a long line of people in the parking lot of Mountain Medical Care Center.

"That looks like a crazy, busy clinic," I said.

"That's a pill mill run by the infamous Dr. Hoover. I can't believe they haven't shut that place down. She's killing people with opioids."

When I returned home, I googled Katherine Hoover, M.D. When she started working for the clinic in 2002, her medical license was suspended. According to West Virginia Board of Medicine records, she had been accused of asking a 17-year-old patient during her first gynecological visit in 1995 if she or any of her friends would "have sex with her teenage sons." She was allowed to continue practicing under the supervision of another doctor.

On Friday I had a full clinic day in Jonesboro, then we saw nursing home patients in the early evening. I returned home late, feeling exhausted. Dr. Kazim was probably about 20 years older than me, and he was like a manic machine! He appeared tireless, happily rushing from place to place to see patients. He was on call 24-7, and he saw patients in two clinics, a nursing home, and two hospitals!

I was thankful I wasn't on call over the weekend. Monday was much more relaxed. I only saw 11 patients in the clinic, and I didn't see any hospitalized patients.

"I'm so hungry!" Dr. Kazim said around noon.

"Well, it is lunch time," I said.

"I'm fasting."

"Oh, yeah. You're going to be fasting all week?"

"Yes."

"You're not going to eat anything at all for the whole week?"

"Yes."

"Okay. I won't tell you how delicious the lunches are." I smiled.

He laughed. "I have the willpower."

On Tuesday I returned to the hospitals. At JMC I saw a new patient, an 86-year-old female with an acute exacerbation of COPD. The lady with the partial diverticulosis perforation had been discharged the day before. Ms. Estep was still in RCH. Her digoxin level had normalized, and she was no longer seeing lightning bugs, but she still had renal failure and lightheadedness.

Tuesday, Wednesday, and Thursday were also more relaxed clinic days, and we saw patients in the Middle of Nowhere, West Virginia, clinic on Thursday afternoon. I continued to see patient after patient with DM, HTN, HLD, and most of them were obese. A 36-year-old morbidly obese female weighed 358 pounds, and her body mass index (BMI) was 57.8. A BMI greater than 30 is considered obese. She complained of shortness of breath, and she had a tracheostomy for obstructive sleep apnea (breathing disruption caused by temporary airway obstruction from excessively bulky pharyngeal tissues). Ms. Estep's kidney function normalized over the days, and she was discharged on Thursday. I saw other hospitalized patients with acute COPD exacerbations, chest pain, CAD, A-fib, and acute pancreatitis.

Friday was a busier clinic day. A 73-year-old female had unexplained weight loss (her BMI had decreased from obese to normal). A chest CT six months earlier showed two lung nodules. A follow-up chest CT three weeks earlier showed a spiculated (spiky) 9x5 mm mass in the right lung, and she was scheduled for a PET scan. A 59-year-old male had a left submandibular swelling, and he was scheduled for a CT and fine needle biopsy. At the end of the day, I congratulated Dr. Kazim for demonstrating his willpower throughout the week.

"Good job," I said. "Are you going to fast this weekend too?"

"No," he said. "I started last weekend. Tomorrow I feast!"

"What will you feast on?"

"Whatever I want. I'll have a big breakfast and maybe some fried chicken for lunch. I'm craving fried chicken."

"How hard has it been?"

"The first few days were the hardest. After that I wasn't hungry until today, when I started craving some delicious, greasy, fried chicken. Maybe I'll have that for breakfast."

"How about fried chicken biscuits?"

"Stop it!"

"You're the one who started talking about it. I like strawberry jam on my chicken biscuits. Have you tried that?" I smiled.

"I am exercising my willpower. I need a drink of water."

Monday was a very busy day. I rushed to both hospitals between 6 and 7 a.m. to see six patients. One of the patients was very ill. Ms. Adkins was 47 years old, and she had sinusitis, nausea, vomiting, hypernatremia (abnormally high sodium), dehydration, fever, leukocytosis (abnormally high white blood cells), and possible meningitis. The result of cerebrospinal fluid (CSF) analysis from a lumbar puncture was pending.

I entered her room. She was asleep in bed with an IV line connected to a bag of normal saline. She appeared obese, older than her stated age, with messy, brown hair.

"Ms. Adkins," I said.

She didn't move.

"Ms. Adkins," I said louder.

She didn't respond, so I gently touched her shoulder, and she jerked awake, startled.

"Who are you! What's going on!" she said.

"Ms. Adkins, I'm James," I said. "I'm a medical student working with Dr. Kazim."

"Okay. Well, I want to see Dr. Kazim 'cause I'm really sick." Her tone was irritable.

"Of course. He will see you soon. Is it okay if I ask you some questions and examine you?"

"I guess. Where am I?"

"Jonesboro Medical Center."

"I don't even remember how I got here."

"What do you remember?"

"I was taking medicine for a sinus infection, but I just kept getting worse, and I felt really sick and started throwing up."

"You do have a fever, and you have a high white blood cell count, which indicates your body is fighting an infection.

You had a lumbar puncture done in the emergency department to check for meningitis, which is an infection of the central nervous system. We're waiting for the result from the lab. Has your neck felt stiff?"

"I feel stiff all over, like all my muscles are tense, and I just can't relax."

"Okay. Could you lie flat on your back?"

She turned onto her back.

I checked for neurological signs of meningitis. I palpated her neck, which felt somewhat tense, and flexed her head toward her chest. Her hips and knees didn't flex, so she had a negative Brudzinski sign. I flexed a hip and extended the knee to check for a Kernig sign.

"Ow!" she said.

"Sorry." I lowered her leg and thigh to the bed. She had a positive Kernig sign, but I thought about how I might have a positive sign, as my right hamstrings were often tight. I checked her knee jerk reflexes, which were abnormally brisk. I auscultated her heart and lungs; the sounds were diminished due to her obesity. Her radial pulse was 116 (tachycardia). I pressed on her abdomen. "Okay. Dr. Kazim will see you soon."

"I'm feeling nauseous again," she said.

"I'm sorry. I'll ask a nurse to get you some Zofran." I handed her a basin.

"Thanks."

I went to a nurses' station. Dr. Kazim soon joined me, and I presented the cases to him.

"Ms. Adkins' CSF lab is pending," I said. "Sinusitis could progress to meningitis, but I'm not sure if she has meningitis. Her neck is a little tense, but I don't think she has nuchal rigidity. Brudzinski sign was negative, but Kernig sign was positive, and she has hyperreflexia."

"Good job with the physical exam," Dr. Kazim said. "But nuchal rigidity and the Brudzinski and Kernig signs aren't reliable. These signs have been used for more than 100 years to help determine if a patient with suspected meningitis needs a lumbar puncture. But according to a prospective study, nuchal rigidity had a sensitivity of 30 percent, and the Brudzinski and Kernig signs each had a sensitivity of 5 percent."

"I didn't know the sensitivities were that low."

"Yes. Let's go see her."

"Okay."

We saw Ms. Adkins and the other patients together. Dr. Kazim decided to continue IV hydration and Augmentin until the CSF lab became available. We rushed to the clinic. I entered the break room for a moment before I started seeing patients. Kevin was eating a pastry, watching CNN coverage of Obama on the TV.

"Good morning," I said.

"Good morning," Kevin said.

"Why don't we see what's on Fox News?" I changed the channel to Fox News.

"Oh, Dr. Kazim won't like that."

I smiled. "Let's see how he reacts."

Dr. Kazim entered the room after a few minutes.

"Good morning, Kevin," Dr. Kazim said, smiling. "Did you actually arrive early today?"

"I did get here a few minutes early," Kevin said. "Are you impressed?"

"Good job," Dr. Kazim said. He poured himself a cup of coffee.

"This pastry is yummy," Kevin said. "Your fast is over now?"

"Yes, but we need to get some healthier food in here, like whole-grain bagels and fruit." He noticed the TV. "Who turned this on Fox News!"

"I don't know," I said. "It was like that when we came in here."

"Yeah," Kevin said.

"We don't watch *Fox News* here!" He changed the channel to CNN, looked at us suspiciously, and we restrained smiles.

"Are your parents in town now?" I said.

"Yes," Dr. Kazim said.

"How's the visit going?" I said.

"Good. Thanks. Okay, let's get to work."

I saw 21 patients in the clinic with all sorts of common problems, but one of the patients had been cursed with a rare problem: Duchenne muscular dystrophy, an X-linked, severe, progressive muscular dystrophy that only affects males. The patient was a 19-year-old male, and he was in a wheelchair due to weakness of his lower extremities. Dr. Kazim prescribed Bactrim for a UTI and refills for omeprazole for gastroesophageal reflux disease (GERD). Dr. Kazim also let me know that Ms. Adkins' CSF was negative for meningitis.

The next day I didn't see Ms. Adkins, but I saw a 50-year-old obese male with type 2 DM who was hospitalized for diabetic ketoacidosis (DKA) after he was noncompliant with insulin. DKA is a life-threatening complication of diabetes that occurs when insulin deficiency inhibits the ability of glucose to enter cells for utilization as fuel, so glucose accumulates in the blood, and the liver compensates by rapidly breaking down fat into ketones for a fuel source. Ketones accumulate in the blood and urine and turn the blood acidic. DKA occurs mostly in patients with type 1 DM but also occurs in some patients with type 2 DM.

"How do we treat DKA?" Dr. Kazim asked me.

"IV fluids, insulin, and potassium," I said.

"Good job."

At the clinic I saw a 50-year-old male with Crohn disease, an inflammatory bowel disease that typically involves the ileum and often spreads to the colon. Crohn disease is characterized by patchy deep ulcers that may cause fistulae (abnormal passages), abscesses, scarring, fever, diarrhea, cramping, abdominal pain, loss of appetite and weight. The patient's disease was stable on sulfasalazine, but the medication sometimes caused nausea, so he also took Zofran as needed for nausea.

I resumed following Ms. Adkins over the next couple of days. Sinusitis, nausea, vomiting, hypernatremia, dehydration, fever, and leukocytosis resolved. Her blood glucose was normal, but she had polyuria (excessive urination) and polydipsia (excessive thirst), and she craved ice-cold water. Dilute urine and random plasma osmolality greater than 295 mOsm/kg suggested a diagnosis of diabetes insipidus (DI), a disease characterized by excretion of large amounts of dilute urine and extreme thirst. DI is caused by inadequate output of pituitary antidiuretic hormone (central DI) or lack of renal responsiveness to the hormone (nephrogenic DI).

"How can we distinguish between central and nephrogenic diabetes insipidus?" Dr. Kazim said.

I pulled out my pocket *Medicine* book from my white coat to find the answer. "Desmopressin test," I said. "Administer 1 microgram subcutaneously and measure urine osmolality at 30, 60, and 120 minutes. Urine osmolality should increase at least 50 percent with central diabetes insipidus and not change with nephrogenic diabetes insipidus."

"Good job. We can also order a water deprivation test."

Dr. Kazim had a rare day off on Friday, so I read about diabetes insipidus. I emailed our rotation coordinator to ask if she had received Dr. Border's evaluation of me, then I enjoyed a nap. Weather was nice for the first weekend of spring: sunny with cool, crisp mornings and high temperatures in the low 70s. Cherry trees and flowers were starting to bloom, grass was turning greener and growing, and some lawns were mowed. I felt my SAD starting to dissipate, and I rode my bike up a mountain to a radio tower behind our apartment.

An upstairs neighbor, a young college guy, also enjoyed the weather by throwing a football behind our apartment. While he was outside, an older man from the end of our building stole a wallet out of his unlocked apartment. Fingerprints from the door matched the thief, who reportedly had hepatitis C and had been in jail multiple times for drug-related charges. He was due in court soon for one of the charges, and another court date was added for theft. I reminded Lynn to always keep our main door locked and keep the piece of wood in the track of our sliding patio door.

On Monday I saw Ms. Adkins again. She had responded to the water deprivation test. Her urine osmolality increased to 307 mOsm/kg (became concentrated). She had also responded to the desmopressin test, but it wasn't clear if she could have CDI or NDI because partial NDI could show a response similar to that seen in CDI. Partial defects in both types of DI occur more frequently than complete defects, so the diagnosis is often complicated. Dr. Kazim decided not to diagnose her with DI, and he discharged her. He said she could have mild DI, but if she did, no treatment was indicated. She would follow up in the clinic for further monitoring.

Thursday was the last and busiest day of the rotation. I saw a total of 31 patients in the Jonesboro clinic and the clinic in the Middle of Nowhere, West Virginia. The last patient of the day was a disabled 32-year-old male, sitting in a chair in an exam room. His right upper extremity was atrophic (had wasted muscle mass), his forearm was contracted and held close to his body, and the skin was pale and cool. He had worked as a coal miner for 11 years, and his right shoulder and humerus were fractured by a falling rock several years earlier. The fractures healed after orthopedic surgery with placement of rods and screws, but he developed reflex sympathetic dystrophy (complex regional pain syndrome).

RSD is a syndrome characterized by pain, swelling, and vasoconstriction of an extremity, and an abnormal sympathetic nervous system reflex, usually following an injury or surgery.

In a healthy person, a sympathetic response to injury causes vasoconstriction to prevent blood loss and swelling. The response soon diminishes, and vasodilation allows for tissue repair. In a patient with RSD, the sympathetic response does not diminish. Prolonged ischemia (deficient arterial blood flow) caused by vasoconstriction worsens pain, and the reflex arc increases the sympathetic response and vasospasm.

"My life has never been the same since that damn rock fell on me," the miner said. "I hate having to depend on the government. A lot of lazy asses around here are happy to cash their disability checks and snort Oxys, but that's not me. I'd rather be working, and I only take Percocet if I really need it. A man is supposed to provide for his family. My dad and grandpa worked in the mines." Tears welled in his eyes.

"I'm sorry," I said.

"Me too. I guess God had other plans for me. Now my wife brings home the bread, and that's hard to accept. I feel useless. I was never depressed before, but now I have to take Celexa."

"Does it help?"

"It helped me to stop thinking about how I'd be better off dead."

"You were really depressed then."

"Yeah, and I wasn't a good father and husband. I've come a long way since then. I've got a good wife and boys." He wiped tears off his cheeks.

"How old are your boys?"

"Twelve and nine. I don't want them to work in the mines. Maybe they can go to college."

"That sounds like a plan. Mining is certainly hard, dangerous work. Is your Celexa working well enough for you?"

"It helps, but I'm still fighting the gloom sometimes, especially when my pain flares up."

"Your dose is 20 milligrams, which is a medium dose. Would you like to try a higher dose if it's okay with Dr. Kazim?"

"Sure. Thanks."

"You're welcome."

Dr. Kazim increased Celexa to a maximum dose of 40 mg. He gave me an excellent evaluation, and I thanked him for the experience. I returned home late, exhausted, and I was thankful to have a three-day weekend before starting my next rotation.

Endnotes

1. FNP: family nurse practitioner.

2. ARB: angiotensin receptor blocker.

3. PA: physician assistant.

4. Renal failure caused an abnormally high creatinine level.

5. Half-life is a measure of the rate of a drug's metabolism and elimination from serum (fluid portion of blood). The digoxin level would decrease by 50% in 1.5 to 2 days.

Chapter 9

Pediatrics

I started my two-month pediatric rotation with Nadia Patel, M.D., in April. My second month was scheduled for November. I was a little apprehensive about seeing children. I had difficulty remembering all of the developmental milestones. Dr. Patel's clinic was also in Jonesboro, Kentucky. She was in a group practice, and her clinic was adjoined to Jonesboro Medical Center. She was an FMG with a medical degree from India, and she had completed a pediatric residency in the U.S.

I arrived at the clinic front desk on Wednesday at 8 a.m., and a female receptionist took me to meet Dr. Patel in her office. On the way I heard a child screaming bloody murder in an exam room. An obese, black woman in scrubs exited the room with two syringes in a hand and shut the door. The child had a set of lungs!

"This is Diana," the receptionist said. "She's one of our nurses."

"Good morning," I said. "I'm James. I'm starting a rotation with Dr. Patel."

"Nice to meet you," Diana said with a smile.

"Those shots must have really hurt," I said.

Diana laughed. "Some children are rather dramatic."

Dr. Patel was sitting at a metal desk in her office, reviewing a paper chart from a stack. She appeared older, petite, wearing a stethoscope around her neck, a yellow blouse, and tan pants. Her white coat was hanging next to her desk on a wooden coat hanger stand. Her office was sparsely decorated, utilitarian. A cheap bookcase next to her desk held some medical textbooks and journals. A golden pothos plant with trailing vines was on a stand below a large window with an open blind.

"Dr. Patel. Good morning," I said. "I'm James Banks."

"Good morning, James," she said with an exotic accent. "Wow, you're tall. Please have a seat."

I sat in a chair in front of her desk.

"How are you?" she said.

"Good," I said. "I enjoyed a long weekend. I had Friday off."

"That's nice. What was your last rotation?"

"Internal medicine with Dr. Kazim."

"Okay. The last student who was with me was planning to become an internist. Do you know Nick? I can't remember his last name."

"Nick Dillard?"

"Yes. How's he doing?"

"He's doing well. He's in the class ahead of me."

"I'm glad he's doing well. I enjoyed having him with me. He did a really good job."

"He's a go-getter. He was a Green Beret before medical school."

"What's a Green Beret?"

"Army Special Forces."

"Really?"

"Yeah. He did special operations in Afghanistan."

"That sounds scary."

"I'm sure it was."

"Please tell him I send my regards."

"I will."

"Have you decided on your specialty?"

"Psychiatry."

"Really?"

"Yeah, as long as I like my psych rotation next month."

"Why psychiatry?"

"It's interesting to me. I just need to make sure I like the clinical aspect of it."

"Where will your rotation be?"

146

"At the psych hospital in Luray."

"That sounds scary too. Are you sure you want to see crazy people?"

"I guess so."

"Okay. Well, our first patient is a 12-year-old girl who's here for her Tdap[1] shot. Let's go see her."

"Okay."

She put on her white coat, and we went to the patient's exam room. The girl was sitting on the exam table, and her mother was sitting in a chair. The girl appeared overweight, with long, messy blonde hair, casually dressed. Her mother was obese, with short, blonde hair, casually dressed.

"Good morning," Dr. Patel said. "This is James. He's a medical student."

"Nice to meet you, James," the mother said.

"Hi," the girl said.

"Nice to meet you," I said.

"How are you?" Dr. Patel said to the girl.

"Okay," the girl said.

"You're here for your Tdap?"

"Yeah."

"You've gained weight since your last appointment, and you actually need to lose weight."

"I know," the mother said. "I've tried to get her to exercise. She just sits around and watches TV or plays on the computer when she's not in school."

The girl rolled her eyes. "You don't exercise."

"I've got a bad back," her mother said.

"What's her diet like?" Dr. Patel said.

"We like McDonald's, but she doesn't eat that much."

"Fast food is full of lots of fat and calories. Is she eating any fruits or vegetables?"

"Aren't fries vegetables?"

"Potatoes are vegetables, but fries are full of fat from the oil they're cooked in. Baked potatoes are a healthier option. Wendy's has baked potatoes and salads, and McDonald's has salads."

"She doesn't like salads."

"What does she drink?"

"She really likes Mountain Dew."

"Oh, that's full of lots of sugar and caffeine, and it causes cavities. How many Mountain Dews does she drink a day?"

"I don't know. She drinks it all day long. We buy the big two-liter bottles 'cause it's cheaper, and they don't last long."

"That's not good. She should avoid sodas and energy drinks, and have only water and milk. If she wants something sweet, she could have a little juice, but it should be 100 percent juice, like apple or orange juice. Juice drinks have very little real juice, and they're full of added sugar."

"Okay."

"Let me have a look at you." Dr. Patel used the light from an otoscope to examine her throat. "She has cavities. How long has it been since she's seen a dentist?"

"It's been a while. She hates going to the dentist."

"How long is a while?"

"Maybe the year before last."

"That's too long. She needs to see a dentist."

"Okay."

"And she really needs to stop drinking Mountain Dew, or her teeth are going to get worse, even if she has good dental care."

"Okay."

The girl had "Mountain Dew mouth," a common condition in Eastern Kentucky caused by excessive soda consumption. In extreme cases, toddler baby teeth rot. Kentucky has the highest percentage of toothless adults under age 65. Dr. Patel examined the girl's ears with the otoscope and auscultated her heart and lungs. Dr. Patel had her lie supine to examine her abdomen, and stand and bend forward, like she was diving, to screen her for scoliosis. Her spine was straight. "Looks good. Diana will be in to give you your Tdap."

"Okay. Thanks, Dr. Patel," the mother said.

"Thanks," the girl said.

"You're welcome," Dr. Patel said.

We left the room and returned to Dr. Patel's office. She wrote a note in the girl's chart, and we went to see the next patient, an 8-year-old girl with vomiting and diarrhea. Dr. Patel diagnosed her with viral gastroenteritis, prescribed Zofran, and advised the girl's mother to use Pedialyte for hydration. She sent me to see the next patient while she completed a note.

Matt was an 18-year-old basketball and football player with an earache, bradycardia, and ventricular bigeminy (premature ventricular contractions followed by normal contractions). Bradycardia by itself is usually normal in athletes with strong hearts. I knocked on the door and entered the room. Matt was sitting in a chair, and he didn't have a parent with him. He appeared tall, handsome, and muscular, wearing an athletic T-shirt and shorts.

"Matt. Good morning," I said. "I'm James. I'm a medical student working with Dr. Patel."

"Hi, James," he said. "Nice to meet you."

"How are you?"

"Okay, except for my ear." He touched is right ear. "It started hurting a few days ago."

"You sound congested."

"Yeah. I've had the crud."

"Have you had a sore throat?"

"No."

"Fever or chills?"

"No."

"And you have bradycardia and ventricular bigeminy?"

"That's what they've told me. I've seen a heart doctor, and he said I could keep playing sports."

"Do you ever get dizzy or lightheaded?"

"Only if I take a hard knock from football, but I shake it off. Sometimes I feel like my heart skips beats."

"Okay. Have a seat on the table, and I'll take a look in your ears."

He sat on the table. I examined his eardrums, nasal cavity, and throat with an otoscope, auscultated his heart and lungs, and palpated his radial pulse.

"Okay. Dr. Patel will be in shortly," I said.

"Thanks," he said.

I went to Dr. Patel's office.

"How's Matt doing?" she said.

"He has an earache that started a few days ago," I said. "He sounds congested, but he denied sore throat, and he doesn't have a fever. It looks like he has clear effusion behind his right tympanic membrane. His nasopharynx appears inflamed and congested. He has some phlegm in his oropharynx, but it doesn't look inflamed. He also has bradycardia and ventricular bigeminy. He denied dizziness and lightheadedness, but he has occasional palpitations. He said a cardiologist has cleared him to continue sports."

"Yes. He has been followed by a cardiologist. No treatment or restrictions were recommended. Let's go see him."

We went to see Matt together, and Dr. Patel examined him.

"You do have some fluid in your right ear," she said. "And you have nasal congestion. You have some phlegm in your throat, but it looks okay otherwise. You haven't had a sore throat?"

"No," he said.

"And no fever or chills?"

"Right."

"Your temperature is normal. Are you allergic to any medications?"

"Not that I know of."

"The fluid in your ear is clear, probably caused by the common cold, which is a viral infection. It doesn't look like a bacterial infection, but it could turn into one, so I'm going to prescribe amoxicillin."

"Okay."

"James said you've also had some palpitations, but you haven't felt dizzy or lightheaded?"

"Right."

"Have you stopped drinking the energy drinks?"

"I've cut back, but I still have a Red Bull or two a day."

"I'm glad you've cut back, but it would be better to have no Red Bulls. Those drinks are full of sugar and caffeine, which is not good for your heart."

"I know. I'm working on quitting. I don't get palpitations as often since I've cut back."

"Maybe you wouldn't have any palpitations if you go ahead and quit."

"I know."

"Okay. I'd like to see you back in a couple of weeks to look at your ear again."

"Okay. Thanks."

"You're welcome."

We returned to Dr. Patel's office, and she took a snack break. She sliced an avocado in half, removed the seed, and seasoned a half with salt and pepper.

"Do you like avocado?" she said.

"Yes," I said.

"Would you like half?" She offered it to me.

"No thanks. I'm not hungry right now. I haven't tried avocado with just salt and pepper. I'll have to try that."

"It's delicious." She started to eat the avocado with a spoon.

"I've used avocados to make guacamole."

"I like guacamole too. How do you make it?"

"Avocados, diced onion and tomato, fresh minced garlic, fresh lime, and a little Kosher salt."

"That sounds delicious. Could you give me the recipe?"

"Sure." I wrote the recipe down on a piece of pocket notebook paper and handed it to her.

"Thank you. I'll give this a try."

We saw a few more patients before lunch: a 10-year-old boy with a scraped knee and hand from a dirt bike accident, a 2-year-old boy with a sty, and an 8-year-old boy for a vaccination. I went to Wendy's and had a baked potato, chili, and side salad, and I returned to the clinic to see more kids with fevers, sore throats, and boo-boos. The first day of my pediatric rotation was a breeze compared to other rotations! During the afternoon while I was in Dr. Patel's office, Lynn called me on my cell phone. We had a quick conversation and decided what we'd have for dinner.

"Was that your wife?" Dr. Patel said.

"Yes," I said.

"You said 'I love you' when you ended the call. I've noticed that married people use this expression a lot in America. Why is that?"

"I haven't thought much about it. My wife and I love each other, so we tell each other. We also tell everyone in our families we love them when we end phone calls and visits."

"My husband and I don't have to say we love each other. It's understood."

"That wouldn't work with my wife. She says she loves me a lot. Was your marriage arranged?"

"Yes, but we love each other. We just don't have to say it all the time."

"Okay."

The next day we saw more kids for vaccinations and kids with sore throats, vomiting, and diarrhea. An 8-year-old obese boy had Mountain Dew mouth. He required a physical before a tooth extraction. The tooth was severely decayed, abscessed, and painful, and his obese mother had finally stopped purchasing soda.

We also saw Levi, a 5-year-old boy who had altered consciousness the previous day. He was sitting on the exam table, and his worried mother was sitting in a chair.

His mother said, "We were eating dinner last night, and he just suddenly stopped talking, and his head went forward like he was going to pass out and hit the plate."

"But he didn't pass out?" Dr. Patel said.

"No."

"How long did it last?"

"Just a few seconds, but it scared me to death."

"Of course. How was he after the episode?"

"Fine. Like nothing had happened. He didn't know he stopped talking in the middle of a sentence, and he couldn't remember what he was saying."

"Okay. He's in kindergarten now?"

"Yes."

"Has his teacher noticed anything with his behavior, like he's sometimes staring off into space?"

"She hasn't said anything, but I can ask her."

"Okay." Dr. Patel turned to Levi. "Let me take a look at you." She examined him and turned back to his mother. "It sounds like he had a near syncopal episode or maybe an absence seizure."

"A seizure!"

"Yes. These types of seizures usually occur in children from age five to nine. Has anyone else in the family had seizures?"

"No. What's a syncopal episode?"

"It's a fainting episode that occurs when not enough blood gets to the brain."

"What causes that?"

"A problem with the heart."

"So he either has a heart condition or something's wrong with his brain?"

"Yes."

"Could he have a tumor in his brain?"

"That is possible but unlikely."

The mother started to cry.

"Don't cry, Mom," Levi said.

"I'm sorry, son," his mother said. "I love you so much!"

"I know, Mom. I love you too."

She hugged him, kissed him on the cheek, and wiped her tears away.

"I'm sorry," Dr. Patel said. "I know this is hard. I will refer him to a neurologist and cardiologist, and the neurologist can order a brain MRI."

"How long will that take?" the mother said.

"Hopefully, they can see you today or tomorrow. I'll give them a call. Why don't you wait here for a little bit, and I'll let you know?"

"Okay." The mother became tearful again.

"I'm sorry." Dr. Patel touched her shoulder, and we left the room.

Both specialists agreed to see Levi during the afternoon. His EKG was normal, and the neurologist scheduled him for an MRI the next day.

On Friday morning while I was seeing a patient, I ignored a call on my cell phone, and I received a voicemail notification. I listened to the voicemail after I saw the patient: "Hello, James. This is Dr. Halper. I expect you're seeing patients now. Please call me back when you can. I need to talk to you about your ob-gyn evaluation."

Alex Halper, D.O., was BCSOM's associate dean of clinical affairs and professor of osteopathic principles and practice (OPP). Dr. Halper taught OPP during my first two years of medical school. He was odd, and he had a talent for twisting students' minds into knots with his lectures and exams. He was older, slim, wore glasses, and he was always clean-shaven and well-dressed, usually wearing a tie.

My heart sank, and I stepped outside the clinic to return the phone call.

"Hello. This is Dr. Halper," he said.

"Good morning, Dr. Halper," I said. "This is James Banks returning your call."

"Hi, James. How are you doing?"

"Well, I was doing fine until I received your voicemail."

"I understand. I'm sorry to have to call you. What rotation are you on now?"

"Pediatrics."

"How's it going?"

"Good so far. Did Dr. Border trash me in my evaluation?"

"It is a bad evaluation."

"I'm sorry. I had a bad feeling about how she was going to evaluate me. That rotation was over two months ago, and I called twice to remind her to complete the evaluation. I think I last called about two weeks ago. Did you just receive the evaluation?"

"Yes."

"How bad is it?"

"Well, she didn't fail you, but in the comments section she wrote that you falsified a medical record for a fundal height exam that you didn't perform."

"I did write down a normal fundal height for one patient without actually measuring because she had a normal ultrasound a week earlier. Dr. Border was very unhappy about that. At the beginning of the rotation, I asked her to recheck a patient's fundal height because I wasn't sure of my measurement, and she acted like I was an idiot and said, 'Did they not teach you how to do that in medical school?' I told her I knew how to do the exam, but the measurement can vary by a few centimeters, depending on where exactly you place the tape measure at the pubic symphysis and where you palpate the top of the uterine fundus. Have you seen my evaluation of the rotation?"

"Yes. I've reviewed that too."

"Okay. Well, practically everything I learned on the rotation I taught myself by seeing patients and reading my ob-gyn book. She did little to no teaching, even when I was inquisitive, and her responses to questions were usually minimal. At the beginning of the rotation, she even said she needed a break from medical students. She acted like she could care less if I was there, and she seemed burned out. Once she threw a tantrum in the OR when a scrub tech handed her the wrong instrument, and she slammed the instrument on the floor. I was so glad when the rotation was over."

"I'm sure you were. Other students have also had problems with Dr. Border."

"That doesn't surprise me. All of my other rotations and evaluations have been good."

"I know you're a good student. This evaluation is an anomaly, but I still need to meet with you to go over the evaluation and discuss this further."

"Okay."

"Can you meet me at my office Monday morning at nine?"

"Yes. I'm sorry, Dr. Halper. I certainly regret not simply pulling out the tape measure for that patient."

"Okay. I'm sorry you had such a bad rotation. I'll see you Monday."

"Okay. Bye."

I went back into the clinic to see more kids. I had difficulty concentrating after the phone call, but I was glad to be busy to keep myself from brooding. Friday was the busiest day of my rotation. I saw 24 patients. I wished I didn't have to wait until Monday to meet with Dr. Halper as it would be difficult to avoid brooding over the weekend. I returned home a few minutes before Lynn. I poured myself a shot of Woodford Reserve bourbon and sank into the couch, feeling very tired and dejected. I took a sip and turned on the TV. An ad for

Eric C. Conn (aka "Mr. Social Security") urged people to call him to "get the disability you deserve."

Lynn entered the apartment and hung up her keys and purse.

"Hey, babe," she said. "I'm so glad it's Friday!"

"Hi, babe," I said.

"Are you okay? Did you have a bad day?" She took off her shoes and sat beside me.

"My day was going fine until Dr. Halper called me this morning. Dr. Border finally completed my ob-gyn evaluation after more than two months, and she trashed me."

"She did!"

"Yes."

"What a bitch!"

"Yeah. And she's a passive-aggressive bitch because she waited for more than two months to trash me."

"How bad is the evaluation?"

"In the comments section, she wrote that I falsified a medical record for a fundal height exam."

"You falsified a record?"

"I wrote down a normal fundal height for one patient without actually measuring because she had a normal ultrasound the week before."

"I remember you telling me about that. You were worried she'd give you a bad evaluation. Did she fail you?"

"Thankfully, no. But I have to meet Dr. Halper Monday morning."

"I'm sorry, babe."

"Me too. I think Dr. Halper will have my back. He said I'm a good student, and other students have also had problems with Dr. Border."

"Big surprise. But if she's had problems with other students, why is the school still allowing students to rotate with her?"

"I don't know."

"You are a good student. Other doctors have given you great evaluations, and you're going to be a great doctor."

"Thanks, babe."

"I mean that. You are going to be a great doctor. I'm so proud of you, and I love you."

"I love you too."

"Dr. Border obviously has issues."

"Yeah. I've thought about writing her a letter."

"No. That would just make things worse."

"I know. I'm not going to write a letter. I just thought about it."

"Good. She goes to our church, and her husband is in the choir!"

"I know, and her husband is really nice. I guess we should avoid eye contact."

"That's probably a good idea. I wouldn't want to give her a piece of my mind and make a scene in church. That wouldn't be very Christian."

"Yeah. That would be bad."

"She's certainly not acting like a Christian. You don't deserve how she treated you. This makes me so mad! What I'd really like to do is slap the bitch!"

"That would definitely be bad."

"Yeah. But she definitely deserves a bitch-slap."

I chuckled.

"I'm serious."

"I know."

"You're going to shake this off and move on. Why don't we order some pizza, get in our comfy clothes, snuggle up, and watch a movie?"

"Sounds good to me."

I was happy to escape into a movie, sex, and sleep. On Saturday I felt depressed, and the gloomy weather matched my mood. I wanted to ride my bike up the mountain behind our apartment to relieve some stress, but rain was falling, so

I sat on the couch and watched TV. Bright green grass and trees popped through the gray outside our patio sliding glass door. I consumed a little too much bourbon over the weekend, and on Sunday Lynn and I studiously avoided eye contact with Dr. Border at the Methodist church in downtown Brighton.

On Monday I met with Dr. Halper in his BCSOM office at 9 a.m., and he reassured me. I wouldn't have to do another ob-gyn rotation, and the school would probably stop scheduling students for rotations with Dr. Border. I returned to the clinic for the rest of the day. Dr. Patel told me she made guacamole from my recipe, and she really liked it. She also told me that Levi's MRI was normal, so his neurologist scheduled him for an electroencephalogram (EEG).

In the afternoon we saw a 10-year-old boy with hereditary spherocytosis, cough, and fever. Hereditary spherocytosis is a congenital defect in the red blood cell membrane that causes the cells to be thickened, almost spheric, fragile, and susceptible to hemolysis (destruction), which results in chronic anemia and mild jaundice. Symptoms from the disease are highly variable, ranging from asymptomatic with mild hemolytic anemia to severe hemolytic anemia with growth failure, splenomegaly (enlarged spleen), and chronic transfusion requirements in infancy necessitating early splenectomy (surgical removal of the spleen). Acute hemolytic crises cause gallstones, fever, and abdominal pain. The boy didn't have abdominal pain, so Dr. Patel suspected that his mild fever was caused by a cold. She ordered a CBC, which showed mild anemia. She advised his mother to give him ibuprofen or Tylenol as needed for fever and to call if his symptoms worsened.

Tuesday was busier, and Wednesday was *very slow*. I only saw four patients, but the first case of the day was heartbreaking. Jonathan was 7 years old, and he was a follow-up for lymphadenopathy (abnormal enlargement of lymph nodes). He was sitting on the table, and his mother was sitting in a chair.

"What happened to his head and neck?" Dr. Patel said. "He has petechiae and contusions."[2] She palpated his cervical lymph nodes.

"He fell down the stairs," the mother said.

"I don't see how a fall down the stairs could cause these injuries. How did he fall?"

"I tripped," Jonathan said.

"Did your mother see you fall?" Dr. Patel said.

"No. She was in the living room."

"Yeah," his mother said. "I was watching TV. I heard him fall, and I ran to see if he was okay."

"Did you take him to the ER?" Dr. Patel said.

"No. He cried for a minute, and he was a little banged up, but he said he was okay."

"Let's take your shirt off." He lifted his arms, and Dr. Patel pulled his shirt off. "He also has contusions on his chest."

"Yeah. He took quite a fall. I'm glad he's okay."

"Does anyone else live with you?"

"My fiancé."

"Okay. Was he there when Jonathan fell?"

"No. He was at work."

"Okay. Is your fiancé Jonathan's father?"

"No."

"How does he get along with Jonathan?"

"Fine, except for when Jonathan gets on his nerves."

"Has your fiancé ever gotten really angry with Jonathan?"

"Jonathan makes me really angry sometimes, and I've given him some good spankings. Sometimes Keith gets angry if he has a little too much to drink, but he doesn't spank Jonathan."

"Keith is your fiancé's name?"

"Yes."

"How long have you been together?"

"On and off for the last few years."

"How long has he lived with you?"

"He moved back in a month or two ago."

"How have you been getting along since he moved back in?"

"We have good days and bad days just like any other couple."

"Okay. Well, Jonathan's lymph nodes feel smaller, and he doesn't have a fever, so that's good. But his injuries are highly suspicious for abuse, so I have to make a report to Child Protective Services."

"Please don't. Keith could go back to jail."

"Keith has been in jail before?"

"It's a long story."

"I fell down the stairs," Jonathan said.

"Please don't make a report," his mother said.

"I'm sorry," Dr. Patel said. "I'm obligated by law to make a report to protect Jonathan."

"Please don't."

"I want to see him back in one month."

We returned to Dr. Patel's office, and she called CPS to report the abuse. According to the U.S. Department of Health and Human Services, Kentucky's child abuse rate was ranked first or second from 2011 to 2018 and in the top 10 from 2008 to 2011. The problem has been attributed to the opioid epidemic, extreme poverty, mental illness and violence in many households, and a chronically understaffed social service system.

Later during our very slow morning, we heard a commotion outside Dr. Patel's office. Dr. Patel quickly went and opened the door at the end of the hall just outside her office, and I followed her. The nurses' station was also near the door, and Diana left the station to look out the door. An older, obese woman was leaving the nearby medical center entrance in a highly emotional state with her hands up in the air, wailing and talking loudly in unintelligible language. We watched her for a moment, Dr. Patel returned to her office, and I closed the door.

"Could you understand anything she was saying?" I said to Diana.

"She's filled with the Spirit," Diana said.

"You mean she's speaking in tongues like a Pentecostal?"

"That's right."

"Someone must have died."

"She'll be alright."

I had never seen a person speak in tongues before!

In the afternoon Dr. Patel let me know that Levi's EEG showed absence seizures, and his neurologist would start him on ethosuximide.

My pediatric rotation was easy, and I liked Dr. Patel. But I soon grew weary of hearing crying and screaming kids, and I became bored. Most of the kids had sore throats, fevers, coughs, ear infections, GI problems, or they just needed vaccinations or well checks. Dr. Patel told me I had good clinical skills, and she couldn't understand why I wanted to become a psychiatrist. Near the end of the rotation, she allowed me to perform OMT on a 16-year-old boy who strained his low back while playing baseball. During my last week we saw a sad case in the hospital: a newborn boy, who was delivered prematurely by emergency C-section due to fetal distress. His mother's urine drug screen was positive for an impressive number of substances: barbiturates, benzodiazepines, opioids, and marijuana. He was initially inconsolable, but he improved over three days. CPS was notified, and he was discharged.

Dr. Patel treated me to lunch in a restaurant with her husband during my last week. Her husband was trim, well-dressed in an Oxford shirt and pants, and he was pleasant. He was a biology professor at a community college. Dr. Patel gave me an excellent evaluation, and I thanked her for the experience.

Endnotes

1. Tdap: tetanus, diphtheria, and acellular pertussis vaccine.
2. Petechiae: small hemorrhages under the skin. Contusions: bruises.

Chapter 10

Inpatient Psychiatry

I was excited to finally start my inpatient psychiatry rotation with Bruce Heimer, M.D., on Friday, May 1. Psychiatry is an oddball medical specialty. Some other physicians don't consider psychiatrists to be "real doctors." Many people, including some physicians, don't know the difference between a psychiatrist and psychologist. A psychiatrist graduated from medical school and completed a four-year psychiatry residency, and a psychologist earned a Ph.D. or Psy.D. degree. Most psychiatrists just provide pharmacotherapy (medication treatment) for patients—even though they learned different psychotherapy modalities in residency—because medical insurance reimbursement rates are higher for pharmacotherapy appointments. Psychiatrists who provide therapy usually have cash-only private practices in affluent areas. Psychologists, licensed counselors, and social workers with master's degrees provide psychotherapy. Unlike other physicians who use patient histories, physical exams, labs, tests, and imaging to make definitive diagnoses, psychiatrists only have patient histories, collateral information, and mental status exams to make diagnoses, which aren't always certain. Psychiatrists have to be comfortable with gray diagnoses.

Dr. Heimer worked at Luray Behavioral Health Center (LBHC) in Luray, a small mining town located one and a half hours from Brighton. Some of the mountains around town had been destroyed by mountaintop removal mining. LBHC was the closest psychiatric hospital to Brighton. It had 96 adult beds, served a 20-county region, and it was adjoined to Luray Medical Center. Both facilities were nice, newer buildings. Dr. Heimer earned his medical degree from the University of Kentucky's

College of Medicine, and he completed his four-year psychiatry residency at the University of Louisville.

I rented a room in a small, three-bedroom house in Luray for $320 for the month so I wouldn't have to commute three hours on weekdays. The landlady lived in Tennessee, and she rented the rooms to medical students. I finished the last day of my pediatric rotation on Thursday, and on Friday morning I left Brighton at 6:15 a.m. to be sure I would arrive at Human Resources in the medical center by 8 a.m. I found my way to HR a little early to complete paperwork and a urine drug screen, which I wasn't expecting. I was glad I hadn't smoked marijuana in a while. Ha ha. I received a key and ID badge that would open locked doors.

I arrived in the LBHC lobby around 9 a.m. to meet Dr. Heimer, and we were the only ones there. The lobby was pleasant, bright with large windows, and well-furnished. Images of nature and Appalachia were on the walls. Dr. Heimer appeared young, trim, handsome, wearing a blue Nike golf shirt and khaki pants.

"Dr. Heimer. Good morning," I said. "I'm James Banks."

"Good morning, James," he said. "Man, you're tall." He firmly shook my hand. "Are you ready to see some psychopathology?"

"Yes. I want to go into psychiatry as long as the crazies don't scare me away."

"Cool. Let's get some breakfast first."

"Okay."

He drove us to McDonald's in his Ford F-150 four-door truck, which had leather seats and a golf bag full of clubs in the back seat. Dr. Heimer drove like he had plenty of time, unlike Drs. Kazim and Coleman. I didn't normally eat breakfast, but I was unusually hungry, so I accepted his offer to buy me two sausage biscuits and a coffee. We ate our breakfast as he drove us back to the hospital.

"Where are you from?" Dr. Heimer said.

"Tennessee. How about you?" I said.

"Kentucky. What got you interested in psychiatry?"

"During my second year a psychiatrist gave us two full days of lectures. He spent half his time working for a VA[1] and half his time teaching for different medical schools. He was really good, and I found the topics really interesting. He said he had a great lifestyle, compared to other doctors, and income for psychiatrists has been increasing with greater demand."

"That's true. I'm working a locum tenens contract here because they have difficulty recruiting psychiatrists and they made me an offer I couldn't refuse. I do have some call, but it's not bad. When I worked in clinics, I had no call and holidays off."

"That sounds good."

"It was, but it didn't fit my financial plan. You should steer clear of working for a VA unless you have a high tolerance for bureaucracy. You have a limited reservoir of energy. Work hard while you're young so you don't have to when you're older. I plan to retire early and play golf. Do you play golf?"

"No, but I like to hike and bike, and I skied and snowboarded when I lived in Colorado."

"I love the West. I have a house on the Oregon coast. I worked for a hospital in Oregon for five years, and I decided to keep the house. It's my castle of solitude."

"That sounds awesome."

"It is. My wife and I spent three weeks there before I started this gig."

"You have a house in Luray too?"

"No. We live in Lexington. I stay here on weekdays, and the locum tenens company pays for my place."

"How do you like Luray?"

"This town is a shithole. Like I said, they made me an offer I couldn't refuse. I can endure a shithole for a hundred fifty an hour. I'm an independent contractor, so I'm not under the thumb of bureaucratic administrators without medical degrees, and I can contribute $49k to my SEP IRA annually. I didn't go through four years of medical school and four years of residency to have pencil-pushing pinheads tell me how to practice medicine."

"You're paid a hundred fifty an hour!" I quickly did the math: $1,200/day, $6,000/week, $24,000/month!

"Yes, and I don't work that hard. Some days I'm done by noon, and I can play 18 holes of golf. Courses are less crowded on weekdays."

"Wow. Maybe I should get a job here after I finish residency."

"The world will be your oyster after you finish residency."

"What's a SEP IRA?"

"A retirement account for a self-employed person or business owner. I'm self-employed as an independent contractor. If I were a hospital employee, I'd only be able to contribute a max of $16.5k to a 403(b) annually. A 403(b) is basically a 401(k) plan for a non-profit organization."

We arrived at LBHC, took an elevator to the second floor, and went to the locked entrance of the 2-East unit. The door had a yellow sign that said, "ELOPEMENT PRECAUTIONS," and a small, thick window at eye level. We could see that no one was in the hall.

"Make sure your badge will open the door," Dr. Heimer said.

My badge opened the electronic lock, and we entered the unit. We walked a short distance down the hall and turned left into the dayroom. It was brightly lit, with large windows and tan walls, furnished with tables, chairs, cushioned seats, and a TV in a corner that was enclosed behind plexiglass. The unit had two long halls on opposite sides of the room. A half dozen patients were in the room, and a male doctor, wearing a long white coat, moved swiftly through the room. He waved to Dr. Heimer and disappeared down a hall.

"That's Dr. Castillo," Dr. Heimer said. "He's another locum doc. He's from Spain."

Several patients approached us as we walked toward the enclosed nurses' station, which had large plexiglass windows facing the room. A middle-aged, disheveled, redheaded woman reached us first.

"Are you going to see me today?" she said to me.

"I'm not sure," I said.

"Dr. Castillo is your doctor," Dr. Heimer said.

"Okay," she said.

"What about me?" said an older, trim, disheveled man with gray hair and a thick beard.

"Yes, Curtis. I'll see you today," Dr. Heimer said.

"Great. I'm ready to go home."

"I don't know if you're ready to go home yet."

"I am. I'm fit as a fiddle."

"You are fit physically, but you need to keep taking your Clozaril for a while longer so you'll be in top mental shape."

"I'm taking the medication religiously, and my mind is sharp, very sharp."

"Okay. I'll talk to you later."

We went to the nurses' station. Dr. Heimer unlocked the door with a key, and we entered the room. Two nurses were sitting at a long desk built into the wall below the large windows, and they were writing in paper charts. They appeared older, overweight, and they were wearing blue scrubs. The whole dayroom was visible through the windows.

"If you don't want patients to bother you as much when you're going through the unit, lose the white coat," Dr. Heimer said to me.

"Okay," I said.

"Good morning, Dr. Heimer," the nurses said.

"Good morning, ladies," he said. "This is James. He's going to help us fix the sad and disturbed souls in here."

"He has his work cut out for him," a nurse said. "I'm Janet."

"Nice to meet you," I said.

"I'm Karen," the other nurse said.

"Nice to meet you," I said.

"They're still sending medical students to you?" Karen said with a grin.

"I have vast knowledge to bestow upon our future doctors," Dr. Heimer said.

"And you're very modest," Karen said.

"I'm confident." He turned to me. "I've been told my personality is too strong, even off-putting, for some of the timid medical students. You don't strike me as timid."

"I don't think you're off-putting," I said.

"Some of the patients find him really off-putting," Karen said. "He received another great review." She pointed to a piece of paper on a bulletin board.

"Read it to me," Dr. Heimer said.

I read the handwritten note: "Dr. Heimer is the worst doctor I've ever seen. I refuse to see him again. I demand to see another doctor who actually cares about his patients. Stacey Hatfield."

"Stacey is a flaming borderline," Dr. Heimer said. "I have a polarizing effect on patients, especially borderlines. They either love me or hate me. What do you know about Clozaril?"

"What's the generic name?"[2] I said.

"Clozapine."

"It's an atypical antipsychotic."

"Okay. What's the difference between atypical and typical antipsychotics?"

"Typical antipsychotics block dopamine receptors. Atypical antipsychotics block dopamine and serotonin receptors."

"What about side effects?"

"Typical antipsychotics have a higher risk of causing tardive dyskinesia.[3] Atypicals can cause metabolic syndrome."

"What is metabolic syndrome?"

"Weight gain, hyperglycemia,[4] hyperlipidemia, and hypertension."

"Okay. What particular life-threatening side effect is clozapine known for?"

"Agranulocytosis."[5]

"Yes. The incidence of agranulocytosis is only one percent, but clozapine requires regular CBC monitoring, so its use is limited. But it's a great medication for treatment-resistant schizophrenia. Have you heard of the rule of thirds for schizophrenia?"

"No."

"A third of patients respond to treatment, a third partially respond, and a third don't respond at all. Curtis isn't responding to a 900-milligram dose of clozapine, which is the maximum recommended dose. He's still psychotic as hell. He's a CIA agent, and he's called in bomb threats to the hospital three times."

"How did he do that?"

"He used the phone in the dayroom. They had to remove the phone."

"What if other patients want to make calls?"

"They have to request the phone. Curtis would be a good candidate for ECT,[6] but, unfortunately, we don't offer that here."

"How long has he been here?"

"Two weeks. Let's go see him." Dr. Heimer grabbed his chart.

"Okay."

We left the nurses' station. Curtis was no longer in the dayroom. We saw him pop out of a room at the end of a hall, run halfway down the hall, throw some nonexistent thing, and run back into the room. We went into the room. It was furnished with two beds, two nightstands, two small desks with chairs, and built-in shelves. Curtis was crouched on the floor with his hands over his ears.

"What's going on?" Dr. Heimer said.

"Get down!" Curtis said.

"Why?"

"I just tossed a grenade!"

"At who?" Dr. Heimer opened the chart binder and started writing a note.

"Gooks."

"Okay. I think you got them. I didn't see them when we came in."

"Are you sure?"

"Yes."

Curtis stood up and peeked into the hall. "You're right. They're gone."

"Curtis, this is James," Dr. Heimer said. "He's a medical student working with me."

"Pleasure to meet you, James," Curtis said.

"Nice to meet you," I said.

"I told James you work for the CIA," Dr. Heimer said.

"I can't talk about that," Curtis said.

"Why not?" Dr. Heimer said.

"It's classified."

"You told me about some operations you did."

"I shouldn't have done that, and no offense, James, but I don't know who you are. I just met you. What medical school are you attending?"

"Brighton College School of Osteopathic Medicine," I said.

"I haven't heard of that school."

"It's in Brighton an hour and a half east of here."

"Okay. What is osteopathic medicine?"

"It's a holistic approach to patient care. The curriculum of osteopathic schools is the same as M.D. schools, except we have additional training in osteopathic manipulative treatment for musculoskeletal problems."

"Interesting."

"Where did the gooks come from?" Dr. Heimer said.

"North Korea. I need to get out of here before they return." He peeked into the hall again. "I'm fit as a fiddle."

"Can you tell James where else you've worked without getting into classified details?"

"Oh, I've been all over the world. Korea, Japan, China, Afghanistan, Iraq, Somalia."

"Wow," I said.

"Yeah. I can say I've been involved in taking out some commies and Al Qaeda terrorists."

"That sounds scary."

"Oh, it was, but our enemies had to be defeated. Dr. Heimer, I'm ready to go home so I can get back to work."

"Like I said earlier, you need to stay here a little longer and keep taking your Clozaril," Dr. Heimer said. "You ended up here because you quit taking your Clozaril again."

"I know. Trust me, I learned my lesson this time. That will never happen again. I will take my medication religiously."

"Okay. We'll see you on Monday."

"My mental acuity is very sharp. I'm thinking very clearly."

"Okay." Dr. Heimer closed his chart.

We left the room and returned to the nurses' station.

"Curtis is obviously crazy as hell, but he's a higher-functioning schizophrenic," Dr. Heimer said. "He's college-educated, and, according to his brother, he actually worked for the State Department years ago."

"Interesting," I said.

"He is an interesting patient. He gets worse every time he goes off Clozaril and decompensates. It takes him longer to recover, and his baseline functioning gets progressively worse, which indicates a poor prognosis. Noncompliance with pharmacotherapy is a common problem in patients with serious mental illness. What are we going to do with him if the Clozaril isn't enough this time, and ECT isn't an option?"

"I don't know."

"We could check a clozapine level and maybe increase the dose higher than the FDA-recommended maximum, or add another antipsychotic, or maybe lithium. What life-threatening side effect would you be concerned about with the use of two antipsychotics?"

"Neuroleptic malignant syndrome."

"Right. What are the signs of NMS?"

"Muscle rigidity, fever, unstable blood pressure, tachycardia, altered mental status."

"Okay. What labs need to be monitored with lithium besides a drug level?"

"Thyroid and kidney function."

"Yes. Why?"

"Lithium can cause hypothyroidism[7] and renal failure."

"Yes. The lithium won't touch Curtis's psychosis, but the medication has a neuroprotective effect, which may help to preserve the brain cells he has left. Why don't we see Stacey next since she's so pleased with the care I've provided? She's 27 years old, and she was admitted after she and her boyfriend boozed it up, got into a fight, broke up, and she cut her wrist. She has a history of superficial cutting, but this laceration required sutures." He grabbed her chart and opened it. A small headshot was in the front of her chart. "She's on Seroquel, lithium, Depakote, and Paxil."[8]

We went to see her. Dr. Heimer spotted her through a window on the balcony, talking to a male patient. We opened the door and stepped onto the balcony, which had a waist-high brick wall and a metal safety grill above the wall to keep patients in. The air was warm and humid. Stacey appeared young, cute, well-groomed, casually dressed. She had long, black hair streaked with purple, tattoos on her forearms, a bandage on her left wrist, and scars on both forearms from prior cuts. The man appeared young, disheveled, with long hair, unshaven, wearing green scrubs.

"Hello, Stacey," Dr. Heimer said. "How are you today?" He opened her chart to start writing a note.

"Fine until now," Stacey said. "Why are you seeing me? I gave a written complaint to the nurses. I refuse to see you anymore."

"Sorry. I'm afraid you're stuck with me until you get out of here. This is James. He's a medical student working with me."

"Nothing against you, James, but I didn't give permission for a medical student to see me."

"I can leave," I said.

"He needs to see patients so he can learn," Dr. Heimer said.

"Well, he shouldn't be learning from you," she said. "I want him to leave."

"Considering your complaint, I insist on him being a witness to our conversation."

"Does a patient not have any rights here?"

The man walked to the balcony door.

"I'll talk to you later, Dustin," she said with a smile.

"Okay." He smiled back, opened the door, and left the balcony.

"I read your complaint," Dr. Heimer said. "Why am I the worst doctor you've ever seen?"

"I'm not suicidal, and I'm ready to go home," she said.

"Okay. Can you tell James why you ended up here?"

"Can he not read that in my chart?"

"Of course he can, but it's good to hear patients' stories in their own words."

"I'm tired of talking about what happened over and over again and being asked the same questions over and over again."

"You said you're ready to go home?"

"Yes."

"Well, I don't usually discharge patients who are hostile and uncooperative."

"I'm sorry. How are you doing today, Dr. Heimer? You're the best psychiatrist I've ever had."

"That's cute."

"I was never suicidal. I had a little too much to drink, and I got really angry with my boyfriend because he was being an asshole. I didn't mean to cut myself that deep. I'm fine now, and I'm taking my medications."

"Have you had any contact with your boyfriend since you've been in here?"

"Yeah. He visited me and said he was sorry."

"Are you back together now?"

"I don't know."

"How long have you been together?"

"A few months. I'm really fine now, and I'm ready to go home."

"Okay. I need to review your nursing notes and see some other patients. I'll let you know about discharge later."

"I'll keep taking my medications and stay away from the vodka. Believe me, I don't want to come back here as long as you're working here."

"I'm glad I can motivate you to avoid another hospitalization."

"I feel sorry for all your other patients. Truly sorry."

We left the balcony and returned to the nurses' station. Dr. Heimer grabbed more charts and handed me a few.

"Let's go to my office. It's easier to talk in there," he said.

"Before you go, could Emmitt get some p.r.n.[9] Ativan?" nurse Janet said. "His anxiety is really bad. He was admitted last night for Xanax withdrawal."

"I'll have to review his chart and see him first."

"Okay. Thank you."

We left the nurses' station and went to Dr. Heimer's office, which was a short distance down a hall. He unlocked the door, and I shut the door behind us. His office was bare. No art was on the walls, the bookcase was empty, and his desk was messy with papers. We set down the charts, and he sat at his desk.

"Have a seat," he said.

I sat in a chair beside his desk.

"Okay. I have three rules for psychiatry," he said. "The staff are sicker than the patients. Don't let the lunatics run the asylum. And don't work harder than the patients work for themselves. What did you notice about Janet's appearance?"

"She's older and overweight," I said.

"She also has bradykinesia,[10] a tremor of her upper extremities, and her affect is restricted."

"Okay."

"She could have Zyprexa-induced parkinsonism."

"What's the generic name for Zyprexa?"

"Olanzapine."

"Okay. That's an atypical antipsychotic. I thought atypicals had a lower risk for causing EPS."[11]

"That's correct, but Zyprexa is very potent, and it's more likely to cause weight gain than other atypical antipsychotics. In any case, Janet frequently asks for Ativan for patients because she's a nervous nurse. She's the one who needs Ativan. Let's take a look at Emmitt's chart and see if he needs Ativan." He opened the chart and reviewed the ED note. "He's 68 years old, and he was taken to the ED by his daughter for altered mental status and panic attacks after he ran out of Xanax 10 days early due to overusing the medication. He doesn't sound like a guy who should get a benzo back. He's on gabapentin 300 mg t.i.d.[12] for withdrawal. We can see him next, but first, let's talk about Stacey. What did you think about her?"

"She's full of drama."

"Yes. Borderlines are definitely full of drama."

"I don't remember all the diagnostic criteria for borderline personality disorder. How do you know if a patient is borderline?"

"After you gain some experience, you'll just be able to smell them after a while."

"Okay."

"I can usually pick up on borderline traits in the first few minutes of an interview."

"Really?"

"Yeah. So should we discharge this borderline patient?"

"Well, she said she wasn't suicidal in the first place, and she was intoxicated with alcohol when she cut herself. You said you want to review her nursing notes. If they're okay, you want to discharge her?"

"I'm asking you."

"Let me take a look at her nursing notes."

"Okay."

I opened her chart and reviewed the notes. "She hasn't been suicidal, and she has been compliant with her medications. She has mostly socialized with male patients. She has been overly friendly with some of them, and she was caught in a male patient's room last night. Maybe that's the guy who was on the balcony with her. Sounds to me like she's ready to be discharged."

"I agree. Borderline crises are short-lived. Borderlines get worse if they stay in the hospital too long. They have splitting behavior, and they create chaos. They should be discharged as soon as possible."

"What's splitting behavior?"

"They treat some staff like they're the best in the world and others like they're the worst. You're either all good, or you're all bad, and their opinion about you can change on a dime. They have black-and-white, all-or-nothing thinking."

"Okay."

"Their lives are typically full of chaos. They have unstable relationships. They often have a history of multiple suicide attempts or self-injurious behavior, and they often have substance abuse disorders, mood and anxiety disorders, and PTSD."[13]

"A lot of drama."

"Yes. There's usually a history of trauma: physical, emotional, or sexual abuse, or neglect. They often end up on ridiculous medication regimens after trying many medications, and managing their medications is a crapshoot. There is no FDA-approved medication for borderline personality disorder, but we can treat their other disorders. Stacey has daddy issues. Her father went to prison for methamphetamine manufacturing when she was a child. She was molested by her older brother and raped by an abusive ex-boyfriend while she was intoxicated."

"That's terrible."

"Yeah. Her mother also had different boyfriends when she was growing up, and she used drugs with her mother."

"That's sad."

"Yeah. Let's go see Emmitt."

"Okay."

We left his office and found Emmitt in the dayroom, watching an X-Men movie on TV with a few other patients.

"Hello, Dr. Heimer," said a middle-aged, disheveled, obese man.

"How are you, Floyd?" Dr. Heimer said.

"I've got these knives in my hands." His speech was monotone, and his affect was flat. He held up his hands, looked at them, and put them back down. He must have thought he could push knife blades out of his knuckles like the X-Men's Wolverine character.

Emmitt appeared older than his 68 years, disheveled, balding, with white hair, unshaven, casually dressed. Dr. Heimer invited him to his office to talk, but Emmitt preferred to just move to a table away from the TV and other patients. He said he took extra Xanax and drank beer because the medication "stopped working" and his "nerves were shot." His anxiety was "through the roof" without Xanax. He pleaded to get back on the medication, and he promised to take it as prescribed. Dr. Heimer increased his gabapentin instead, and, of course, Emmitt was very unhappy.

"We have to get to a meeting," Dr. Heimer said.

We grabbed charts from his office and went to a conference room in the other hall. He unlocked the door with a key. We entered the room, and I shut the door behind us. We sat at a long table with nurse Karen and three other women. Dr. Heimer introduced me to the social worker, psychologist, and utilization manager. We discussed the cases and their treatment plans. I was a little distracted by the psychologist. She was a sexy blonde, and I had to consciously avoid looking at her too much. The utilization manager said that Dr. Heimer needed to do a "doc-to-doc" phone call with Curtis's medical insurance company to discuss the medical necessity of continuing hospitalization, and she pointed out the cases without medical insurance. We left the room after the meeting and headed to the medical center for lunch in the cafeteria.

"I hate doc-to-docs," Dr. Heimer said. "They're such a waste of time. I have to talk with a sellout who works for the insurance company to explain why a patient needs to stay in the hospital longer. Sometimes, the slimeballs deny more hospital days, and sometimes I lose my cool with them. An insurance doctor isn't liable if I discharge a patient prematurely, and they hurt or kill themselves or someone else. I never let a patient's finances affect my clinical judgment. I really don't care what the utilization manager has to say. I'm not going to run discharge all the patients without insurance. I'll discharge them when it's appropriate, and I'll prescribe cheap, generic medications they can afford. When they're in the hospital, I don't have to worry about wasting my time with doc-to-docs."

We enjoyed a leisurely lunch and saw several more patients with substance abuse disorders. Two of the patients were diagnosed with polysubstance dependence, a disorder that is in the American Psychiatric Association's Diagnostic and Statistical Manual of Mental Disorders Fourth Edition (DSM-IV) but not the DSM-5. Patients with polysubstance dependence use at least three different substances (not including nicotine and caffeine), and they have no drug of choice. They use whatever they can get their hands on with reckless disregard for their lives.

The first day of my inpatient psychiatry was very interesting. When I was in the 2-East unit with crazy people all around me, I felt like I was in the middle of a scene from a movie, like *One Flew Over the Cuckoo's Nest*. And I liked it! I made the 1.5-hour drive back to Brighton and arrived home after Lynn. We enjoyed a leisurely weekend, and on Sunday afternoon I packed a bag to stay at the house in Luray during the week.

"I don't want you to go away," Lynn said.

"I know, babe," I said. "I'll call you every night, and I'll be home on Friday night."

"I know, but we've never been apart this long before."

Lynn was especially snuggly on Sunday evening. We watched a movie, had sex, and fell into a deep sleep. On Monday morning we hugged and kissed before I left at 6:30.

"I love you," Lynn said.

"It's understood," I said.

"That's not funny. I'm not Dr. Patel. I said I love you."

"I love you too. I'll call you tonight."

"Okay."

I arrived at LBHC at 8 a.m. and saw new admissions with Dr. Heimer. One of the new admissions was Mr. Sadler, a 53-year-old male with severe depression, suicidal ideation, Crohn disease, and arthritis. Depression had worsened because his declining physical health made his quality of life miserable, and he had his brother take his guns when he started thinking about suicide again. He had attempted suicide in the past by gunshot wound to his chest, and he barely missed the heart and aorta. It was easy to empathize with him. Dr. Heimer prescribed Zoloft and lithium, and he explained that lithium has an antisuicidal effect.

I started following patients. Curtis approached me as soon as he saw me enter the dayroom. He had drool on his thick beard.

"How are you this fine morning, sir?" he said.

"Good. How are you?" I said.

"What's your name again?"

"James."

"James, I feel great. Could you put in a good word for me with Dr. Heimer, and let him know I'm ready to go home today?"

"I can let him know, but I think he wants you to stay here a little longer. Did you see any more Koreans over the weekend?"

"No."

"Good."

"Yeah. I'm glad they're gone. Those commie bastards are evil. Pure evil."

"Dr. Heimer will see you later."

"Okay. I'm good to go."

Floyd still had knives in his hands, and I couldn't get him to say much more than that. Emmitt's anxiety was still "through the roof" without Xanax, and he wanted to be discharged so he could resume the medication from his primary care doctor.

I left the dayroom and headed to an addict's room. As I was walking down the hall, an older, disheveled, obese woman popped out of her room, glared at me and said, "I despise you!" I froze, waited for a moment, and she went back into her room. I cautiously continued down the hall and saw a 36-year-old female with polysubstance dependence and substance-induced mood disorder. She was withdrawing from Ativan, and she was depressed and anxious.

I met Dr. Heimer in the nurses' station, and we saw the patients together. Emmitt was discharged, and the discharge summary would be sent to his primary care doctor so he would be aware of the Xanax overuse and hospitalization. Floyd was also discharged, even though he was delusional, because he wasn't an imminent danger to himself or others.

On Tuesday Dr. Heimer decided for Curtis to try an antipsychotic combination (Abilify was added to Clozaril). On Wednesday we saw a 48-year-old male with schizophrenia vs. substance-induced psychosis. He was using methamphetamine prior to hospitalization, and he had an impressive history of 10 years of methamphetamine use and eight psychiatric hospitalizations. He was paranoid and delusional, thinking people were after him and monitoring him with cameras and other devices. Dr. Heimer prescribed Haldol.[14]

"His brain is fried," Dr. Heimer said after we saw him.

On Thursday the addict was discharged. On Friday Curtis was still floridly psychotic, Mr. Sadler was still severely depressed and suicidal, and the meth head's brain was still fried. I was happy to return to Brighton on Friday afternoon. I was the only medical student staying in the small three-bedroom house, so I was lonely during the week, even though I had phone conversations with Lynn every night. We really enjoyed each other's company over the weekend since we missed each other, and we had especially hot sex.

On Monday I saw more patients with polysubstance dependence, substance-induced mood disorder, benzodiazepine withdrawal, and schizophrenia. The meth head's paranoia was better, so he was discharged. Curtis was still crazy as hell, and he still wanted to be discharged so he could "get back to work." Mr. Sadler was a little less depressed, but he felt like he wasn't quite ready to go home. On Tuesday he was no longer suicidal, so he was discharged. I saw a 56-year-old female with bipolar disorder and psychogenic polydipsia (excessive fluid consumption caused by psychiatric disorders), which caused severe hyponatremia (blood sodium level less than 125). Her sodium level was 124, and she was confused and lethargic with slurred speech. Hospital staff had to watch her closely to keep her from drinking out of sinks and toilets. She was sneaky though. Her sodium dropped to 121 on Wednesday, so she was transferred to the medical center for treatment. Severe hyponatremia can cause seizures, delirium, coma, and sudden death.

On Thursday I saw Amy, a 32-year-old female who was admitted involuntarily for bizarre behavior and homicidal threats. We had pages of neatly handwritten notes about her history from her mother and a copy of a neuropsychological evaluation that had been done three years earlier. Her maternal grandmother had paranoid schizophrenia and spent many years in a psychiatric hospital. Amy received counseling for a few months after the neuropsychological evaluation, but she was never treated by a psychiatrist, and she was on no medications. She had been unemployed for four years, and she previously worked as a computer programmer after she earned a bachelor's degree in computer science. She had no friends or interest in having friends. Her parents often heard her laughing hysterically in her bedroom or bathroom, and she denied laughing when asked why she was laughing. She often became agitated, screamed at her parents, and told them to get out of "my house." She didn't recognize her sister and sister's husband when they visited. She sometimes didn't recognize her father, and she asked her mother why she brought a "strange man" into "my house." She believed that her parents were part of a Mexican drug cartel, and she was a NASA astronaut who had visited Mars.

She sought excessive medical treatment for the past three and a half years, insisting that various symptoms were from serious, undiagnosed medical problems. This behavior started with her visiting an ER 11 times during a two-month period, complaining of severe abdominal pain. Medical workups were negative. During one visit the doctor told her she was just having a normal menstrual period, but she demanded "real tests" to be "properly diagnosed." A psychiatrist evaluated her, diagnosed her with hypochondriasis, and recommended outpatient follow-up. She refused to leave the ER until "real tests" were done, and she demanded to see a "real doctor." Hospital security had to be called, and police escorted her out of the ER. Six months later a psychologist conducted the neuropsychological evaluation with a battery of intelligence, cognitive, emotional, and personality tests, and he diagnosed her with pervasive developmental disorder not otherwise specified (atypical autism) and schizotypal personality disorder traits.

Three days before admission Amy's mother was watching TV near midnight, and she had the volume low to avoid disturbing anyone. Amy "stormed out of her bedroom," turned the TV off, and shouted, "I'm just going to have to KILL YOU if you don't get out of my house!" She grabbed her purse and shouted, "I'm going to a hotel, and you better not be here when I get back!" She left the house, didn't return until the following afternoon, and she didn't mention the incident. A month earlier she told her parents that people were walking down their road with guns, and she demanded for her parents to stop them. Her parents explained that one neighbor walked down the road with a cane, and the other neighbor carried a big stick to keep dogs away. Amy said, "Well, I'm just going to have to GET A GUN and stop them myself!" She went to Walmart to buy a gun, but she didn't have enough money.

Dr. Heimer and I led Amy to his office, and he allowed me to conduct the interview for her admission psychiatric evaluation. She appeared her stated age, obese, disheveled, with light brown hair, wearing green scrubs. Her affect was flat.

"How are you this morning?" I said.

"I want to go home," she said. "I don't understand why I'm here."

"Your parents were really concerned about your behavior."

"What did they say about my behavior?"

"Your mother said you threatened to kill her if she didn't get out of your house."

"That's a lie."

"So you haven't had any homicidal thoughts?"

"No."

"What about suicidal thoughts?"

"No."

"Why do you think your mother would say such a thing?"

"I have no idea. We don't get along well."

"Is your mother in your house?"

"We do live together."

"Do you own the house?"

"The house is paid for."

"Okay. Did you pay for it?"

"What does the house have to do with why I'm here?"

"According to your mother, you have been screaming at her and your father and telling them to get out of your house."

"The house is paid for."

"Okay. Did you see people with guns walking down your road last month?"

"Yes."

"Did you go to Walmart to buy a gun to stop them?"

"No. I just went to get some stuff I needed."

"Okay. Do you think your parents are part of a Mexican drug cartel?"

"They're mixed up in something. They're loaded with cash."

"Have you seen them with large amounts of cash or drugs?"

"No. But I know they have lots of money. Dad bought a brand-new Cadillac."

"Okay. Did you go on a NASA mission to Mars?"

"I can't talk about classified missions."

"Okay. You used to work as a computer programmer. Why don't you do that anymore?"

"That was a long time ago. Everyone I worked with was weird, so I quit."

"Did you look for another job?"

"No."

"Why not?"

"Everyone was weird, and I just couldn't work with weird people again. My parents kept nagging me to find another job, but then I got sick."

"What happened to you?"

"I had debilitating stomach pain, and I saw a bunch of doctors, but they all said they couldn't find anything wrong with me."

"Is that when you visited an ER 11 times in a two-month period?"

"I don't know if I went that many times. I was just trying to get a diagnosis."

"According to your mother, police had to escort you out of the ER during one of your visits."

"That's a lie."

"Okay. Did you ever get a diagnosis after the ER visits?"

"Unfortunately, no. Something's wrong with me, but my doctor can't figure it out. I need to find a specialist."

"Why do you think you need to see a specialist?"

"I think I have a brain tumor. I've been getting bad headaches, bad dizzy spells with blurry vision, and I've almost passed out and fallen. I've had problems talking and thinking, and I've had nausea, numbness, and tingling in my arms and legs, and I've been really weak."

"Have you had your head scanned?"

"Yeah. I had a CAT scan a while back. But I need an MRI. Can I get an MRI while I'm here?"

"Sorry," Dr. Heimer said. "We don't have an MRI machine here. You'll have to ask your primary care doctor about that."

"He won't order it for me," she said. "Can you send me to the medical center to get it done?"

"I'm sorry. You can't leave here right now. James needs to ask you some more questions."

"Okay," she said.

"Have you ever had surgery?" I said.

"No. But I may need surgery if I ever get properly diagnosed."

I asked more questions to complete the interview, and Dr. Heimer took over.

"I think you need some Risperdal," he said.

"What's Risperdal?" she said.

"It's a medication that can help you think and talk more clearly."

"What kind of medication is it?"

"It's an antipsychotic."

"You think I'm psychotic?"

"I think you're having problems with your thoughts and emotions, and you haven't been getting along well with your parents. The medication can have a calming effect and help you get along better with your parents."

"I don't need an antipsychotic. I just need to go home."

"Well, I'm going to prescribe the medication, and you can refuse it, but I recommend you take it if you want to go home."

Dr. Heimer opened the door, and Amy left his office.

"She's a good case for you to see," Dr. Heimer said. "It looks like she has a very unusual blend of autism, schizophrenia, and somatization disorder, or hypochondriasis. Talk about psychopathology!"

Somatization disorder is a mental disorder characterized by a history of extreme focus on many physical complaints in the absence of a known medical condition. Patients with somatization disorder (somatic symptom disorder in the DSM-5) think the worst about their symptoms and seek excessive medical care, searching for an explanation even after serious conditions have been ruled out. Health concerns can become a central focus of life and significantly impair functioning.

On Friday Curtis was a little less crazy and "fit as a fiddle" after taking Clozaril and Abilify for 10 days, and Dr. Heimer increased Abilify.

During my third week Curtis was finally fit enough to be discharged after being in the hospital for more than four weeks. Amy was still refusing Risperdal, and she had an involuntary hospitalization court hearing. A non-treating psychiatrist, who evaluated her for a second opinion, agreed that she needed antipsychotic treatment, so the judge issued court-ordered treatment. Dr. Heimer told her she could take the Risperdal pills or get injections of the medication. She didn't like needles, so she reluctantly agreed to take the pills.

I also saw another patient who was admitted involuntarily for bizarre behavior. Adam was a 24-year-old schizophrenic who had been admitted to LBHC several times over the past two years for psychotic, disorganized, and catatonic behavior after he was noncompliant with medications. Adam's outpatient psychiatrist offered a long-acting injectable antipsychotic to improve his compliance, but he refused.

Catatonia is a rare psychomotor disturbance that can occur in people with psychotic and mood disorders and other medical conditions. Catatonia is commonly characterized by stupor — inability to move, speak, or respond to external stimuli while apparently being awake — but some people may have agitation and excessive movement. Other symptoms include catalepsy (waxy rigidity of limbs, which remain in whatever position they are placed), waxy flexibility (slight, even resistance to positioning by the examiner), negativism (opposition or no response to instructions), posturing (spontaneous and active maintenance of a posture against gravity), stereotypy (frequent repetition of the same, typically purposeless movement, gesture, posture, or vocalization), echopraxia (repeating the movements of others), and echolalia (repeating the words of others). Catatonia can last from a few hours to weeks, months, or even years.

According to Adam's father, he was talking to people who weren't there, and his boss fired him from his handyman job because he was running into things with equipment, forgetting things, wandering off projects, having weird behavior, working with only one hand, holding his water bottle all day, standing on one leg, swatting and throwing nonexistent things, laughing for no reason, losing touch with reality. He became overly religious, drove to his girlfriend's house and read her a passage from the Bible. When he attended church several weeks earlier, he pretended to shoot people with an imaginary gun, and he ducked behind a pew like he was avoiding return gunfire. He said he thought he was in a video game, and he rode home with his head out of the window and tongue out.

Dr. Heimer and I led Adam to his office, and I interviewed him. He appeared his stated age, with short, red hair, unshaven, wearing green scrubs. He had bradykinesia, and he sat erect with his hands on his knees. His affect was flat.

"How are you this morning?" I said.

"It's morning?" he said.

"Yes."

"Oh. It did look light outside through the windows, but I just thought the moon was really bright." He laughed oddly. "What day is it?"

"Wednesday."

"Okay. I had no idea what day it is. I don't know where I am either, but it seems like I've been here before."

"You're in Luray Behavioral Health Center."

"Okay. I thought this place looked familiar. I have been here before."

"Yes. You've been here several times. Do you know why you're here this time?"

"I think I took some drugs."

"Why do you think you took drugs?"

"I feel like I'm tripping, like I took LSD."[15]

"What else do you think you took?"

"I'm not sure."

"Why aren't you sure?"

"I don't know."

"When do you think you took the drugs?"

"It doesn't matter. The drugs should be out of my system by now. I could drive home, but I really need to get back on my Geodon."[16]

"How long have you been off Geodon?"

"For a while."

"How long is a while?"

"I don't know. Maybe three to four months."

"Well, let's get you back on Geodon then," Dr. Heimer said.

"Yes, doctor," he said stiffly. "I will take my medication."

"Good."

I asked more questions to complete the interview, and Adam left Dr. Heimer's office.

During my last week a nurse caught Amy cheeking a Risperdal tablet, so Dr. Heimer switched her to Risperdal M-Tabs (orally disintegrating tablets). The last interesting patient I saw was Mr. McCracken, a 59-year-old disabled male with a history of anxiety and depression who was admitted for suicidal ideation with a plan to overdose. He had pages of handwritten notes, detailing many symptoms, and a typewritten page of 28 medications he had tried! He had taken Xanax, trazodone, Remeron, Lamictal, Wellbutrin, propranolol, Valium, Ativan, BuSpar, Paxil, Abilify, Seroquel, Klonopin, Geodon, Zoloft, Prozac, Zyprexa, Saphris, benztropine, hydroxyzine, Pristiq, Risperdal, Lexapro, Cymbalta, Celexa, Effexor, amitriptyline, and lithium.

Dr. Heimer and I led Mr. McCracken to his office, and I interviewed him. He appeared older than his stated age, balding, with a very thin, sandy blond comb-over, clean-shaven, wearing green scrubs. He was very tremulous, and he was hyperventilating. His affect was highly anxious.

"How are you doing?" I said.

"I'm *terrible!*" he said between breaths. "That's why I'm here. I think I'm having a nervous breakdown! I really need help! My psychiatrist doesn't know what else to do with me, and I'm at the end of my rope!" He sobbed dramatically.

"I'm sorry you're feeling so bad."

"Thank you."

"You've been having suicidal thoughts with a plan to overdose?"

"I don't think I could actually ever go through with it. I don't want to go to hell."

"You believe suicide is morally wrong?"

"Yes. I'm a Christian."

"Do you attend a church?"

"Yes."

"Okay. Tell me why you've been feeling so terrible."

"I'm just having panic attacks and anxiety and depression *real bad!*" He continued to shake, hyperventilate, and he sobbed again.

"What are your panic attacks like?"

"Oh, they're *horrible!* My heart feels like it's going to beat out of my chest, or I'm going to have a heart attack. I get dizzy, my arms go numb, and I feel like I'm going to pass out. I can't catch my breath, and I feel like I'm going to *die!* I throw up in the mornings."

"That sounds miserable."

"It is! It's unbearable! And I've had diarrhea too."

"How long have you been vomiting and having diarrhea?"

"For the past two to three months. My psychiatrist had me try propranolol and Lamictal[17] because Xanax wasn't helping, but they made me really nauseous, and I was throwing up more, so I quit taking them."

"Have you vomited since you stopped the medications?"

"Yes. I've still been vomiting every morning, so I don't know for sure if the medicines were making me sicker."

"Are you still taking Xanax?"

"Yes. I've been taking it four times a day. It's helped a little bit, but it's not strong enough, and my doctor won't increase it."

"You've also taken Valium, Ativan, and Klonopin before. Did any of those medications work better?"

"No. They didn't help at all. That's why I'm on the Xanax. It's the only thing that works for my nerves."

"Okay. Have you used alcohol or any illegal drugs?"

"No, sir. I've never been a drinker or used anything illegal, and I take my Xanax exactly as it's prescribed."

"Okay. And you've also been taking Remeron and trazodone?"[18]

"I've been taking trazodone, but I had to stop Remeron because it was giving me bad nightmares. That was the last medicine my doctor had me try. He hoped it would help with my sleep and appetite and nausea."

"How long do your panic attacks last?"

"All day long!"

"Wow. I've never heard of panic attacks lasting that long before."

"Well, they used to just last 15 to 30 minutes, but then I started having attacks back to back, and lately they've been lasting all day."

"When did your attacks start getting worse?"

"They've been getting worse and worse over the last few months until I just couldn't take it anymore."

"How often have you been having the attacks?"

"*Every single day!* And I get *no relief!*" He sobbed. "Please help me! I need relief!"

"Of course. How long have you felt depressed?"

"I'm always depressed, but that's been worse lately too. It's been *so bad*. I just lay in bed, but I can't sleep, and I hear things that aren't really there. I can't eat. I have no energy."

"What sort of things have you heard?"

"I've heard my phone ringing, knocking on my door in the middle of the night, my name being called."

"That must have been scary to hear a knock on your door in the middle of the night."

"It was! It was *very scary*. I was afraid to answer the door. I looked through the peephole, and no one was there."

"What else have you recently tried for depression?"

"I tried that dang Wellbutrin, but it was *horrible*, so I only took it once. It made me feel like I took acid. The walls were moving, and I was seeing purple colors and halos."

"Did you ever take acid in the past?"

"No. I never touched that stuff. I never even tried marijuana."

"You've tried quite a few other antidepressants: Paxil, Zoloft, Prozac, Pristiq, Lexapro, Cymbalta, Celexa, Effexor."

"All those medications made me feel weird."

"Has anything been stressing you out recently?"

"My mom drives me crazy."

"Do you live with your mother?"

"No. I live with a good friend. He takes medications too, but he's not nearly as bad as me. He helps to calm me down."

"That's good that you have a supportive roommate."

"Oh, yes. He's wonderful. I don't know what I'd do without him."

"Do you work?"

"Oh, no. I wish I could work, but I'm not able to. I'm still scared to drive."

"How do you support yourself?"

"I'm on the draw."

"You're on disability?"

"Yes."

"How long have you been on disability?"

"About 10 years."

"Have you had psychotherapy?"

"Yes. I saw my therapist the week before last. She's wonderful. She helps me a lot. She's shown me breathing exercises, but my panic attacks are just out of control."

"You've tried a lot of medications," Dr. Heimer said. "Do you want to increase Xanax?"

"Yes, please! That would be wonderful! I just need some relief from this terrible anxiety!"

I asked more questions to complete the interview, and Mr. McCracken left Dr. Heimer's office.

"Wow," Dr. Heimer said. "I feel drained, even though you did his evaluation. Talk about histrionic! He should join the local theater."

The next day Mr. McCracken was less anxious and no longer suicidal, so he was discharged. On Thursday the executive director of LBHC met with me because she heard that I planned to become a psychiatrist. She gave me a written offer for a job, which was unexpected and exciting, considering that I hadn't even graduated from medical school. The offer looked very attractive with a great salary, a signing bonus, and a $1,500 monthly stipend, which I would receive during my four-year residency in return for four years of service at LBHC after completion of residency. I showed the offer to Dr. Heimer after the meeting.

"Don't take the bait," Dr. Heimer said. "The money looks great to a poor medical student. That's how they get you on the hook. But what if you sign a contract and take all that money, then you decide in residency that you want to be an outpatient psychiatrist? What if you come back here to work, and you're miserable, but you're locked into a four-year contract? Financial penalties for breaking the contract would be steep. How do you think you and your wife would like living in Luray for four years?"

"I don't think we'd want to live here," I said.

"Like I said, this town is a shithole. Why do you think they're throwing money at medical students? They can't recruit and retain staff psychiatrists, and locum tenens docs like me are expensive. You'd be a great deal, compared to me, if you sign that contract, and they'd have you by the balls for four years. Wait until your fourth year of residency to look for your first job. Recruiters will be after you. You'll get better offers, and you'll be able to take your pick. The world will be your oyster."

"Thanks for the advice."

"Sure. Residency will be miserable enough, especially in the first two years. When you're done, you should be happy and making plenty of money to buy a nice house and car and pay off those student loans as soon as you can. And if you don't like a job, you should be free to leave."

On Friday I thanked Dr. Heimer for the experience. He gave me a glowing evaluation, his cell phone number, and email address, and he encouraged me to contact him if I had any questions or needed advice. Amy was still in the hospital when I left.

Endnotes

1. VA: Veterans Affairs Medical Center.

2. During my second-year pharmacology course, only generic names of medications were used. During my third year I had to add brand names to my vocabulary.

3. Tardive dyskinesia: involuntary movements of the facial muscles, tongue, torso, and limbs that develop after prolonged antipsychotic use.

4. Hyperglycemia: abnormally high blood glucose.

5. Agranulocytosis: an acute, potentially lethal condition characterized by a severe decrease in white blood cells; infected ulcers are likely to develop in the throat, intestines, and skin.

6. ECT: electroconvulsive therapy.

7. Hypothyroidism: diminished production of thyroid hormone, which causes a low metabolic rate, weight gain, and lethargy.

8. Seroquel: antipsychotic. Lithium: mood stabilizer. Depakote: antiepileptic mood stabilizer. Paxil: serotonergic antidepressant/ antianxiety medication.

9. p.r.n.: abbreviation for Latin phrase, meaning as needed.

10. Bradykinesia: slow movement.

11. EPS: extrapyramidal symptoms (abnormal movements).

12. t.i.d.: abbreviation for Latin phrase, meaning three times a day.

13. PTSD: Posttraumatic stress disorder.

14. Haldol is a first-generation antipsychotic.

15. Lysergic acid diethylamide (LSD) is a potent hallucinogen.

16. Geodon is an antipsychotic.

17. Propranolol is a beta blocker that is used off-label for anxiety. Unlike other beta blockers, it crosses the blood-brain barrier to calm down the sympathetic ("fight-or-flight") nervous system. Lamictal is an antiepileptic mood stabilizer.

18. Remeron and trazodone are sedating antidepressants.

Chapter 11

Outpatient Psychiatry

I did my elective outpatient psychiatry rotation with Robert Damron, M.D., in June at Mountain Behavioral Health Services (MBHS), a community mental health center in Brighton. MBHS was in an older, three-story building, and the second floor, where Dr. Damron saw patients, was dim and depressing, like a tired government facility. Dr. Damron was a graduate of the University of Louisville's School of Medicine. He completed three years of a psychiatry residency and a two-year child and adolescent psychiatry fellowship, and he saw kids and adults.

Dr. Damron was young and fit, with a neatly trimmed beard, and he always looked fashionable and professorial, wearing Ray-Ban Wayfarer eyeglasses, Oxford shirts, and chino pants in a range of colors. He had effeminate mannerisms, and he looked at me in a way that made me a little uncomfortable. He told me he had broken up with his partner, and he was thinking about moving to Charleston, South Carolina. Brighton was certainly not a gay-friendly town. He also told me his HIV medications cost $1,200 per month.

Aside from making me a little uncomfortable, Dr. Damron was very nice and happy to have a student with him. I sat next to him as he saw patients in his cramped office. He wrote notes in paper charts and wrote paper prescriptions. He discussed cases and DSM criteria with me, and he treated me to lunch at a greasy diner.

He was out of town for two days, so gave me two journal articles to read about treatment of comorbid depression and anxiety, and coadministration of tramadol and antidepressants increasing risk of serotonin syndrome and seizures. Tramadol is a mild opioid that also weakly inhibits reuptake of neurotransmitters serotonin and norepinephrine into presynaptic nerve cells, which increases levels of the transmitters in the synaptic cleft for binding to postsynaptic nerve cell receptors. Antidepressants also increase serotonin and norepinephrine levels. Excessive serotonin levels can cause serotonin syndrome, which is very similar to neuroleptic malignant syndrome and can be fatal.

I saw plenty of patients with Dr. Damron, and most of them had major depressive disorder and generalized anxiety disorder. I was glad to have the community mental health experience, but it quickly became boring. I thanked him for the experience, and he gave me a great evaluation.

Chapter 12

Medical Detoxification

I did my medical detoxification rotation with Joseph Nichols, M.D., in July when the days were turning hotter and humid. I didn't care for sweltering summer weather. I looked forward to the cooler, drier days of autumn. Dr. Nichols was a family physician who worked in Brighton Medical Center's eight-bed detox unit for alcoholics and addicts. The unit and patients' rooms were small, dingy, and gloomy. Dr. Nichols was older, slim, wore glasses, and he was always clean-shaven and well-dressed. He had a pleasant manner, and he enjoyed teaching. Unfortunately, there wasn't much to learn on the rotation, which was required by BCSOM.

Almost all of the patients were diagnosed with polysubstance dependence, and they stayed in the unit for three to five days if they didn't leave prematurely against medical advice. They all received phenobarbital (a sedating barbiturate), clonidine (a calming antihypertensive) if their blood pressure wasn't too low, and comfort medications. I asked Dr. Nichols why he used phenobarbital, instead of a benzodiazepine, which was used much more commonly for detox. He said that patients didn't enjoy phenobarbital like benzos, so the medication didn't reinforce addictive behavior. He didn't want patients coming into the unit with the ulterior motive to just get benzos.

I enjoyed having more free time during the rotation, especially since I was doing practice questions to prepare for the COMLEX Level 2-Cognitive Evaluation, which I was scheduled to take during the rotation. The exam was computer-based and contained 400 multiple-choice questions, divided into two four-hour sections. I answered sets of 50 practice questions in 60-minute sessions, and I completed about 1,500 questions as I did to prepare for the COMLEX Level 1, which also had 400 questions. The Level 2 exam was as grueling as the Level 1. I felt good about my performance, and I returned to the detox unit the next day.

I quickly became bored with the rotation, and I had little patience or empathy for the addicts. I thanked Dr. Nichols for the experience, and he gave me a good evaluation.

Chapter 13

Consultation-Liaison Psychiatry

I was excited to start my visiting consultation-liaison psychiatry rotation with Thomas Anderson, M.D., during the last week of July. Consultation-liaison psychiatry (also called psychosomatic medicine) is a subspecialty of psychiatry that focuses on the care of patients with comorbid psychiatric and general medical conditions. Dr. Anderson was the assistant program director for the University of Northeast Tennessee psychiatry residency, which I was interested in attending. Dr. Anderson was an American who had attended a Caribbean medical school, and he had completed psychiatry residency at UNT.

On Sunday evening after dinner, Lynn and I hugged and kissed, said we would miss each other, and I made the two-hour drive south to Hansen to stay with friends for the rotation. Lynn and I planned to see each other on weekends, alternating visits between Hansen and Brighton. I arrived at Hansen Medical Center (HMC) on Monday at 7:45 a.m. HMC was a 440-bed teaching hospital that was affiliated with UNT's medical school. Students, residents, and fellows in 14 different specialties and subspecialties worked in the hospital. I took the elevator to the top seventh floor and went to the small medical student coordinator's office. The office had free drinks and snacks! After I completed paperwork and received a badge, I sat in front of a computer to familiarize myself with the EMR.

Dr. Anderson had given me his cell phone number. He sent me a text message, saying he was on his way, and he met me a few minutes later. He entered the office energetically with a bright smile on his face. He appeared middle-aged, slim, handsome, clean-shaven, wearing a blue Oxford shirt and khaki pants.

"Good morning, Judy," he said to the student coordinator just inside the entrance.

"Good morning, Dr. Anderson," she said. "How are you?"

"I'm doing great! How about you?"

"I'm okay. I could use some of your energy. Maybe I need another cup of coffee."

"I like my Starbucks."

"Dr. Anderson, good morning," I said, standing to meet him. "I'm James Banks."

"Welcome, James," he said, shaking my hand. "You're a tall guy too. How are you?"

"I'm good, thanks."

"Have you done everything you need to do here?"

"Yes."

"Good. Let's go downstairs. I need some coffee and a bite to eat."

We went to the doctors' lounge on the first floor. The lounge was nice, well-furnished, and had hot and cold breakfast foods and beverages, including Starbucks coffee.

"Help yourself," he said. "A resident and a couple of other students will meet up with us shortly."

"Okay. I'll have a coffee," I said.

He got a coffee and bagel, and we sat at a table.

"Where are you from?" he said.

"Tennessee," I said. "How about you?"

"Albuquerque."

"Well, you're a long way from home."

"Yeah. But I like it here. What got you interested in psychiatry?"

"During my second year a psychiatrist gave us two full days of lectures. He was really good, and I found the topics really interesting. I enjoyed my inpatient psych rotation in May, and I did an outpatient psych rotation in June."

"Cool. You should be ready to hit the ground running then. Why are you interested in our program?"

"My wife and I like Hansen. We met and got married here just before I started medical school."

"Cool. So you're going to be a D.O. We haven't had a D.O. in our program before."

"Well, maybe I'll be the first."

"Maybe. So you know how to crack bones?"

"I did learn HVLA, which is a high velocity low amplitude technique, but I prefer gentler techniques. I don't like to crack bones, especially in the neck. During my second year a neurologist discussed a case of vertebral artery dissection that was caused by chiropractic treatment. The patient had a cerebellar stroke and all kinds of neurological deficits."

"What a terrible case."

"Yes."

"Well, I like the osteopathic holistic philosophy. My wife's doc is a D.O., and she really likes him."

"Cool."

Kazi Chiranjeevi, M.D., and two medical students came into the lounge. Dr. Chiranjeevi was an FMG with a medical degree from India. He appeared young, clean-shaven, and he and the other students were wearing white coats.

"Kazi, good morning," Dr. Anderson said.

"Good morning, Dr. Anderson," he said with a thick, exotic accent. "This is Laura and Tyler."

"Welcome," Dr. Anderson said, standing to shake hands. "This is James. He's a visiting student."

"Nice to meet you," I said, standing and shaking hands.

Laura was a sexy, curvaceous Latino with long, black hair, who spoke English as a first language. Tyler was a skinny, kind-looking guy with curly, brown hair.

"Do you all want to grab a coffee and something to eat before we hit the floors?" Dr. Anderson said.

Dr. Chiranjeevi and the students got some food and coffee and sat at the table with us.

"How many consults do we have today?" Dr. Anderson said.

"Five so far," Dr. Chiranjeevi said.

Laura said she was going into psychiatry, and Tyler said he was going into family medicine.

"So you're going into psychiatry too!" Laura said to me.

"Yeah," I said.

"Cool!" She smiled brightly and touched my arm. "I'm so excited to be starting this rotation."

"Me too," I said.

"Do you know how to do osteopathic manipulation?" she said.

"Yeah," I said.

"Cool. I have a friend who's going to a D.O. school. So if I get a kink in my neck, you can loosen me up?"

"Sure." I figured it would be a lot of fun to get really loose with her, but I was happily married.

After we finished breakfast, we all went to see the first patient together.

Dr. Chiranjeevi presented the case to Dr. Anderson just outside the patient's room: "Ms. Coke is a 64-year-old African American female who was first seen by Raj two days ago. She was admitted one week earlier for severe COPD, and she developed progressive respiratory failure and pneumonia requiring intubation. Nursing staff reported that she has had altered mental status since admission. She had been petting her IV line and sucking on it. She threatened to kill a nurse, and she said the nurse was having an affair with her sister-in-law and smoking crack cocaine outside her room. She became belligerent and agitated, hit staff, and tried to bite them. She was placed in four-point restraints and given point five milligrams of Risperdal prior to Raj seeing her, and she was not arousable for interview. She is also on Xanax point five milligrams t.i.d.,

Lortab, clonidine, Solu-Medrol, Combivent, levofloxacin, insulin, carvedilol, lisinopril, Lasix, sodium chloride, potassium chloride, and Lovenox. Raj diagnosed her with delirium, MS Contin[1] withdrawal, rule out substance-induced psychotic disorder, and he recommended point two five milligrams of Risperdal q.a.m., point five milligrams q.h.s.,[2] and point two five milligrams daily p.r.n. for agitation. According to the MAR,[3] she has been compliant with her medications."

Dr. Chiranjeevi knocked on the door.

"Come in," Ms. Coke said.

We entered the room. Ms. Coke was sitting up in bed with breakfast on a tray in front of her. She had an IV line, and she wasn't wearing her oxygen line. She appeared older than her stated age, disheveled.

"Well, I must be special," she said. "I've got a whole team of doctors."

"Ms. Coke, good morning. I'm Dr. Chiranjeevi."

"Dr. who?" she said.

"You can call me Dr. C."

"Okay."

"This is Dr. Anderson, my attending, and we have medical students with us: Laura, Tyler, and James."

"Nice to meet all of you," she said.

"How are you doing today?" Dr. Chiranjeevi said.

"Okay. I'd like to go home."

"You'll have to ask your other doctor about that. We are with the psychiatry consult service."

"Psychiatry! Why am I being seen by psychiatry! I'm not crazy!"

"We were consulted because you had some behavioral issues over the weekend."

"Seriously? Who said I had behavioral issues?"

"Do you mind if I have a seat?"

"Go ahead."

Dr. Chiranjeevi sat in a chair next to her bed. "According to staff, you were petting your IV line and sucking on it—"

"What! I did no such thing!"

"You also threatened to kill a nurse, and you said the nurse was having an affair with your sister-in-law and smoking crack cocaine outside your room."

"You must have me mixed up with someone else!"

"Your name is Louise Coke, date of birth March 7, 1945?"

"Yes, but I did no such things. I have been known to raise my voice and speak my mind, but I am not a violent person."

"Okay. Well, you did become combative and hit staff, and you tried to bite them. You were put in restraints to protect yourself and others, and you were given Risperdal to help calm you down."

"I am not a violent person."

"Okay. Well, you have been very ill and delirious. You were hospitalized for severe COPD, and you had to be put on a ventilator for respiratory failure and pneumonia."

"I remember why I came to the hospital, but it's been a blur since I was put on the breathing machine."

"Right. Well, delirium is a condition that affects the brain and causes confusion, disorientation, altered consciousness, agitation, and hallucinations."

"Hallucinations? You mean like seeing things that aren't really there?"

"Yes."

"Well, I haven't had any hallucinations. Like I said, I'm not crazy."

"Okay. So you have no history of mental health treatment?"

"No."

"Your chart indicates you had withdrawal from MS Contin. What were you taking the medication for?"

"I've had pain ever since I had chemotherapy for breast cancer."

"When did you have chemotherapy?"

"That was four or five years ago."

"Okay. Have you used alcohol or any other drugs that aren't prescribed to you, like cocaine?"

"I used cocaine back in the day, but that was over 20 years ago. I have a glass of wine every now and then."

"Okay. Have you had any suicidal or homicidal thoughts?"

"Like I said, I'm not a violent person. Life is a gift from God."

Dr. Chiranjeevi asked her orientation questions. She didn't know the day, date, or floor she was on, but she knew the month, year, season, city, state, and name of the hospital.

Dr. Anderson moved closer to her bed. "Thanks for talking with us," he said. "I'm sorry you ended up in the hospital. That must have been scary when you had to be put on the ventilator."

"It was. I thought I was going to die," she said.

"Well, I'm glad you're feeling better." He smiled charismatically and touched her arm. "We'd like to check on you again tomorrow if you're still here."

"Okay. Thank you." She smiled.

"You're welcome," Dr. Anderson said.

I noticed a stark contrast between Dr. Chiranjeevi's and Dr. Anderson's bedside manners. Dr. Chiranjeevi was a robotic data gatherer. Dr. Anderson was an empathic human, and he made the patient smile.

We left the room, closed the door, and Dr. Anderson discussed the case in the hall.

"Delirium is a common problem in the hospital, and it's associated with increased morbidity and mortality. Some patients still have symptoms of delirium one year after discharge. The mortality rate for patients admitted with delirium is up to 25 percent, and it's up to 75 percent for patients who develop delirium during hospitalization. Aside from illness and MS Contin withdrawal, what else could have caused her delirium? This is a question for the students. Let's look at her medication list."

Dr. Chiranjeevi pulled up her medication list on a computer that was on a high, built-in desk next to the patient's door, and we reviewed the list.

"Benzodiazepine withdrawal could cause delirium if she was off her Xanax," Laura said.

"Good," Dr. Anderson said. "What else?"

We were silent for a moment.

"What about Solu-Medrol?" Dr. Anderson said.

"A steroid can cause delirium?" I said.

"Yes. She could have had steroid-induced psychosis. Steroids can make people crazy. Who's next?"

We saw several older patients with dementia, delirium, and a younger patient with bipolar disorder. Dr. Chiranjeevi was paged several times for more consults, and we saw the rest of the patients in the afternoon without Dr. Anderson. One patient had polysubstance dependence, and another patient had adjustment disorder (depression and anxiety due to a brain tumor in the frontal lobe). Dr. Chiranjeevi told us about the last patient in the hall before we entered her room.

"Ms. Pitts is a 22-year-old female," Dr. Chiranjeevi said. "She is a frequent flier we know well. She has mood disorder not otherwise specified, borderline personality disorder, and she has repeatedly been admitted for ingesting all sorts of things. She has swallowed razors before, but she didn't remove the protective packaging from the razors. This time she ingested batteries and pearls, and she had an EGD to remove the foreign bodies."

"Wow!" Tyler said.

"She is a very difficult case. She has a history of trauma: physical and sexual abuse. She is on a polypharmacy regimen with Trileptal, Abilify, Prozac, BuSpar, Vistaril, and Klonopin, and she has tried many different psychiatric medications." Dr. Chiranjeevi knocked on her door.

"Come in," Ms. Pitts said.

We entered the room. Ms. Pitts was sitting up in bed, wearing a hospital gown. Her knees were bent, and she had a coloring book on her thighs and a crayon in her right hand. She appeared her stated age, with green hair, multiple piercings in her ears, eyebrow, nose, and lip, and she had tattoos on her forearms.

"Ms. Pitts, good afternoon," Dr. Chiranjeevi said. "Do you remember me? I saw you a few months ago when I was on call."

"Sure, but I can't remember your name," she said.

"I'm Dr. Chiranjeevi."

"Oh, yeah. Dr. C."

"I have some medical students with me. This is James, Laura, and Tyler."

"Nice to meet all of you," she said.

"How are you feeling?" Dr. Chiranjeevi sat in a chair next to her bed.

"I'm okay, thanks. I'm ready to go home."

"You were hospitalized again for swallowing objects. This time you swallowed batteries and pearls. Were you having suicidal thoughts before you did this?"

"No."

"Did you know that battery ingestion can kill you?"

"Yeah. But I wasn't suicidal."

"You knew that swallowing a battery could kill you, but you weren't suicidal?"

"Yeah."

"Why did you swallow the objects then?"

"I don't know. I just did."

"Were you upset before you did this?"

"No more than usual. I'm tired of living with my parents. I need to find my own place."

"Have you looked for your own place?"

"Yeah, but I don't want to live in a Section 8 dump that has bed bugs, meth heads, and drug dealers. I can't afford a decent place with my disability check."

"Were you taking your medications before you were admitted?"

"No. They weren't working, so I quit taking them."

"How long were you off your medications?"

"Two or three weeks."

"Have you been following up with Dr. Clark at New Horizons?"

"Not for a while. Dr. Clark is a jerk. He just talks to me for, like, five minutes and pushes pills. He doesn't really care about what I have to say. I need to see a different doctor."

"Okay. Well, it's important to take your medications. They probably help you more than you realize."

"Yeah. When I was off the meds, I was having crazy mood swings, and I was going off. I know I need to stay on them now."

"Good. Do you have a therapist?"

"Yeah, but she's not helping me either."

"Has she discussed coping skills with you?"

"Yeah. But she wants to talk about my past trauma, and that just makes me feel worse."

"Well, that actually indicates you have discussed important issues during therapy. You may feel bad after the sessions, but working through trauma would be good for your mental health in the long run."

"Yeah. Well, I don't want to feel bad when I'm having a good day. I just have to take things one day at a time. I can be fine one day but terrible the next, and I can have a great day suddenly turn to shit."

"I understand. Well, I'm not recommending any medication adjustments for you. I simply recommend for you to remain compliant with your medications and follow up with First Horizons. We'll check on you again tomorrow if you're still here."

"Can you tell my doctor I'm ready to go home?"

"Sure, but your doctor may want to keep you here a little longer to make sure you don't have any complications from swallowing batteries."

"Okay. Thanks."

"You're welcome."

We left the room. Dr. Chiranjeevi asked each of us to pick a patient to see for follow-up the next day, and we could write notes in their paper charts. The charts were like BMC's charts. Doctors' illegible progress notes and orders were handwritten in paper charts, and the EMR contained vitals, labs, imaging, dictated reports, and medication lists. Tyler picked a 77-year-old female with delirium, dementia, and hypothyroidism; Laura picked Ms. Pitts; and I picked Ms. Coke.

On Tuesday morning Laura, Tyler, and I saw the patients together. Laura was an enthusiastic bundle of energy. She moved close when she talked to me and touched my arm at times. She wasn't wearing a wedding ring, and she wasn't touchy-feely with Tyler. Tyler's patient didn't know what was going on when he awakened her. Prior to admission she hadn't seen a doctor in decades, and her family finally convinced her to go to the hospital for worsening auditory and visual hallucinations. A thyroid lab panel showed hypothyroidism, and she was started on Synthroid (synthetic thyroid hormone) and low-dose Seroquel for hallucinations. Ms. Pitts hadn't tried to swallow any more objects, and she was still ready to go home, especially since a nurse had been such a "bitch." Ms. Coke hadn't tried to assault staff again, and she was also still ready to go home. Drs. Anderson and Chiranjeevi met up with us, and we saw all of the patients together.

After lunch Laura and I attended a residents' meeting in a basement room of the old Veterans Affairs (VA) outpatient psychiatry building. The room was cramped, had a low ceiling, and the air was cool and musty, but the room wasn't entirely oppressive. It was well lit, and it had several small, fogged windows at the top of the exterior wall that let some natural light in. Residents and attending psychiatrists sat around a long conference table, which didn't have enough room for everyone, so some sat along the walls, including me. A PowerPoint presentation was projected on a wall-mounted screen at one end of the room. Dr. Anderson introduced Laura and me to some residents, attendings, and program director Bali Vaswani, M.D. Dr. Vaswani appeared older, obese, with a red dot on his forehead, wearing a white Oxford shirt and navy pants. Most of the residents were also Indian.

"So both of you want to be psychiatrists?" Dr. Vaswani said with an exotic accent. His eyes were wide, and his eye contact was intense.

Laura and I said, "Yes."

"What's wrong with you!" he said, looking at us incredulously.

We were taken aback. I said, "Uhhh—"

"I'm just messing with you," he said, laughing heartily. "Seriously, though, you've got to be at least a little crazy to go into psychiatry, right? I've been told I'm crazy and weird, but I embrace my craziness. So, James, you're from Tennessee, and you're attending a D.O. school in Kentucky?"

"Yes," I said.

"Well, we've never had a D.O. in our program before. How would licensing and board certification work for you in an M.D. program?"

"After my first year of residency, I would take the COMLEX Level 3 to get my medical license, and I would be eligible to take the M.D. psychiatry board exam after I finish residency."

"Okay. Very good. What do you think of the C-L[4] rotation so far?"

"Dr. Anderson is great, and we've already seen some interesting cases."

"I agree," Laura said.

"Good, good. Dr. Anderson is great, isn't he? That's why I made him my right hand man. He just finished our program and started the C-L rotation. Well, we've got to get started."

Dr. Vaswani started the meeting by discussing some residency issues, then another Indian attending gave a short presentation about schizophrenia. After the presentation a variety of Psychiatry Resident-in-Training Exam (PRITE) questions were projected onto the screen for residents to answer and discuss. The PRITE is a 300-question exam that most residency program directors in the U.S and Canada use to assess the competence of their residents and the effectiveness of their educational programs. I was happy to correctly answer a question about Tegretol, an antiepileptic/mood stabilizer used to treat bipolar disorder.

Laura and I left the meeting together.

"What did you think of Dr. Vaswani?" I said.

"I think he has good insight because he knows he's weird," she said.

I laughed. "Yeah, he's weird. And he looked kind of crazy with those big eyes."

"I know, right?"

"Are you planning to apply to this program?"

"Yeah, but I think I want to go to the University of Virginia. Dr. Anderson is cool, but this program doesn't have a great reputation, and the residents aren't happy."

"Why is that?"

"I think didactics are lacking, and residents are used as slave labor for the VA."

"Really?"

"Yeah. The VA basically owns the residency program."

"I noticed most of the residents are Indians, and they all looked so serious. I think Dr. Vaswani is the only one who smiled."

"Exactly. Better programs don't have FMGs, or they don't have many of them."

"Well, thanks for the inside information. I was hoping to move back to Hansen. I know residents are indentured servants, but I wouldn't want to be a miserable slave for four years."

"Exactly."

When we returned to HMC on Wednesday, we followed up with Tyler's delirious, demented, old lady, but Ms. Pitts and Ms. Coke were no longer in the hospital. Laura decided to follow a 63-year-old female with alcohol dependence and depression, and I decided to follow a 97-year-old female with delirium, dementia, and a UTI. She was just *old*! Thursday was a short, easy day. Our three patients were the only ones to see. On Friday Laura's patient was gone. My very old lady was still demented, and Tyler's patient's hallucinations had improved. We saw other patients with depression, anxiety, dementia, psychosis, and opioid dependence. And we saw Ms. Carson, a 77-year-old black female with catatonic schizophrenia.

Prior to hospitalization Ms. Carson had been off Risperdal Consta (long-acting injectable antipsychotic administered every two weeks) for one month. According to nursing staff, she hadn't eaten or spoken a word for two days. Labs were significant for elevated creatinine (due to renal failure), elevated creatine kinase (due to muscle damage), and normal serial troponins (no heart muscle damage). A CT scan of her head showed no acute intracranial abnormalities. Ms. Carson was sitting up in bed, blankly staring ahead. She appeared older than her stated age, thin, heavily wrinkled, wearing a hospital gown, and she had an IV line connected to a bag of fluid. A younger black man was sitting in a chair next to her bed.

"Ms. Carson. Hello. I'm Dr. Chiranjeevi with the psychiatry consult service, and I have some students with me."

She remained still and didn't respond.

"What's your relation?" Dr. Chiranjeevi said to the man.

"I'm her son."

"Okay." Dr. Chiranjeevi turned to the patient. "Ms. Carson, how are you?"

She didn't respond.

"She's been like this for a few days," her son said. "She stopped talking and eating. She was diagnosed with schizophrenia a long time ago, and she's had episodes like this before. She sees a doctor at New Horizons."

"Okay. And she's been off Risperdal Consta for a month?"

"Yeah. She missed a couple of appointments for injections, and I didn't know she missed the appointments until she got sick. She lives by herself, and I check on her. But I work, so she has a friend drive her to her appointments, or she takes the bus."

"How was she doing before she was off the medication?"

"She was okay. She hears voices all the time, and she's heard Jesus, but she manages okay when she's on her medication. I knew something was wrong when I kept calling her, and she didn't answer the phone. So I went to her apartment, and I had to get her landlord to let me in 'cause she wouldn't answer the door. When I got in there, she was standing in the middle of the kitchen, frozen, staring into space. She had wet her pants, and I couldn't get her to say a word. I called the clinic to find out what was going on, and I took her to the hospital."

"Okay. Ms. Carson, I need to examine your arms and legs."

She didn't respond.

Dr. Chiranjeevi waved his hand in front of her face, but he didn't faze her trance. He palpated the muscles in her upper extremities, flexed her forearms, and she kept her forearms in the position after he let go. He palpated the muscles in her lower extremities and flexed her hips and knees. He moved her forearms back down to the bed.

"She has catalepsy," Dr. Chiranjeevi said. "We'll start her on IV Ativan for catatonia and hold Risperdal until CK[5] normalizes."

"Okay. Thank you, doctor."

"You're welcome."

On Friday afternoon Laura, Tyler, and I headed out of HMC together.

"Well, I think the first week of C-L was cool," Laura said.

"That catatonic patient was quite interesting," Tyler said.

"Very interesting," I said.

"I hope I get to follow a different patient next week," Tyler said.

"Are you getting bored with the demented, old lady?" I said.

"Yeah." Tyler parted from us in the parking lot to head to his car. "Well, have a good weekend."

"You too," Laura and I said.

Laura turned to me. "Hey, I'm having some friends from med school over to my place tonight for food and drinks. You wanna join us?"

"Thanks for the invite, but my wife's coming into town tonight," I said.

"Well, she can come too." She touched my arm.

"Okay. I'll ask her, but she'll probably want to hang out with our friends tonight. Let me get your number, and I'll let you know."

We exchanged phone numbers, went to our cars, and left. I called Lynn and let her know about the invite.

"So a chick from medical school invited you to a party?" Lynn said.

"She invited you too," I said.

"Uh-huh. What does she look like?"

"She's fat and ugly."

"Uh-huh. Maybe we should just stop by the party so I can tell her to stay away from you."

"That would be hard for her to stay away from me since we're on the same rotation."

"You know what I mean."

"I know. I figured you'd want to hang out with Brian and Helen, and that's fine with me. I just said I'd let you know about the invite."

"Well, you can tell her that you and your *wife* will be spending the evening with our friends."

"Okay, babe."

"Don't forget who's putting you through medical school."

"You're my one and only, babe."

"I better be because if you ever cheat on me—"

"I know. You'll be homicidal."

"And I might pull a Lorena Bobbitt on you."

"Well, I certainly wouldn't want that to happen. I love you and look forward to seeing you."

"I love you too, and I really miss you. I'll leave as soon as I get off work. I'm all packed up."

"Good. Drive safely."

"Okay. Bye."

I sent a text message to Laura to politely decline her invitation. Lynn arrived at 7 p.m., and we enjoyed the weekend with our friends. She told me to watch out for Laura before she departed on Sunday afternoon.

When I returned to HMC on Monday at the beginning of August, Derek Rogers, M.D., an American resident, was starting the C-L rotation. He appeared young, overweight, clean-shaven, wearing glasses, a yellow polo shirt, and navy pants. Tyler was relieved that his demented, old lady was gone. Ms. Carson's catatonia had improved over the weekend, according to medical progress notes and nursing reports. Laura and I wanted to interview her, but we agreed that Tyler should have a turn with an interesting patient.

Ms. Carson was sitting up in bed, watching TV. A tray of eaten breakfast food was on the table beside her bed. She didn't have an IV line, and her son wasn't in the room.

"Ms. Carson. Good morning," Tyler said. "We're medical students with the psychiatry team. I'm Tyler, and this is James and Laura."

"Well, hello there," Ms. Carson said. "You're a fine-looking team."

"Thanks. How are you today?"

"Well, I'd be better if I was home. I hate hospitals. Can you tell my doctor I want to go home?"

"Of course. Do you know why you ended up in the hospital?"

"I was told I got sick again because I was off my medicine. I didn't mean to miss my appointments. I guess they just slipped my mind. I just thought I was in some crazy dream. I saw Jesus."

"You saw Jesus?"

"Yes."

"What did he look like?"

"He was wearing a bright, white robe that was glowing like light, and he was handsome with dark hair and a beard. He told me not to worry because all things work together for good for those who love the Father and are called according to his purpose. I felt a sense of peace like I've never felt before."

"Your son told us that you hear voices, and you've heard the voice of Jesus before."

"Yes, honey. I have schizophrenia, and I hear Jesus from time to time."

"Are you hearing voices now?"

"Yeah. I hear my voice and your voice." She laughed.

Tyler smiled. "I appreciate your sense of humor."

"Well, I'm glad I could make you smile. You look so serious. But you have a nice smile."

"Thanks."

"I mean it. You shouldn't hide that smile."

"Okay." Tyler smiled. "So since you've been in the hospital, have you heard other voices besides yours and mine?"

"Yeah. I've heard nurses and doctors." She smiled.

Tyler smiled. "You know what I mean."

She laughed. "Yeah. The other voices come and go. I need to get back on my Risperdal, or they'll get worse."

"Okay. Your Risperdal has been held because your CK lab showed some muscle damage. You were catatonic before you were hospitalized. Catatonia can make your muscles rigid and can cause muscle damage. Your CK has been going down though. We'll talk with the resident and attending psychiatrist, and they'll see you too."

"Okay. Thank you."

"You're welcome. It's good to see you talking and joking. When we saw you on Friday, you weren't talking, moving, or eating."

"Yeah. I've had these episodes before."

Drs. Rogers and Anderson agreed that it was okay to restart Risperdal. Ms. Carson received oral Risperdal, a Risperdal Consta injection, and she was discharged.

We saw the rest of the patients with the doctors. A 21-year-old female with polysubstance dependence and substance-induced mood disorder had overdosed, and her drug screen was impressive—positive for benzodiazepines, marijuana, cocaine, and opioids. I followed her over the next couple of days, and she was discharged.

During the rest of the week, we saw a number of other patients who overdosed with different substances and prescribed medications. A 42-year-old female overdosed with alcohol, Seroquel, Wellbutrin, Effexor, BuSpar, Cogentin; and a 52-year-old male overdosed with Aggrenox, Flomax, lisinopril, Aricept, Cymbalta, trazodone. We also saw a 42-year-old male who had a suicide attempt vs. an accident. His story was that he was changing a light bulb in a ceiling fan. He used a box cutter to remove a screw because he didn't have a screwdriver, and he fell and accidentally cut his abdomen. Fortunately, the laceration wasn't deep enough to involve the peritoneum, so closure of the wound was uncomplicated. We were skeptical of his story, of course, but he was alone when the incident happened. He had no known history of mental illness, alcohol, or substance abuse, and his blood alcohol level and urine drug screen were negative. He gave us permission to obtain collateral information from his girlfriend, and she corroborated his story. So Drs. Rogers and Anderson told him to buy a screwdriver, and he was discharged.

During my third week Dr. Anderson assigned a new consult to me on Tuesday afternoon. I would conduct the initial psychiatric evaluation by myself and present the case in the morning. The psychiatry team would see the patient together, discuss assessment and plan, and Dr. Rogers would dictate the official psychiatric evaluation for her chart.

"She looks like a tough case, but I think you can handle it," Dr. Anderson said with a smile.

Ms. Flores was 38 years old, divorced, and she was admitted for left lower lobe pneumonia with left pleural effusion that caused shortness of breath, difficulty breathing, and sharp chest pain. Pleural effusion, also called "water on the lungs," is excess fluid between the two layers of pleura that line the outer surface of the lungs. Ms. Flores had been started on IV antibiotics, and she was on a slew of other medications for DM, HTN, HLD, diabetic neuropathy, migraines, fibromyalgia, bipolar 1 disorder, and PTSD. Fibromyalgia is a chronic disorder characterized by widespread pain, tenderness, and stiffness of muscles and associated connective tissue that is typically accompanied by fatigue, headache, and sleep disturbances.

Ms. Flores' medication regimen included *nine* medications that act on the central nervous system (CNS)! Her psychiatric regimen included Seroquel, Paxil, Xanax, trazodone, and prazosin; and other CNS medications included Topamax (antiepileptic) for migraines, gabapentin for neuropathic pain and fibromyalgia, Percocet for chronic pain, and Flexeril for muscle spasms. She also had borderline personality disorder, which was apparently flaming, so I was leery of seeing her. She had been admitted two days earlier, and she wasn't getting along well with all the nurses and doctors. According to her chart, she had been "hostile, verbally aggressive, cursing, demanding, entitled." She refused to allow certain nurses to check her vitals, administer medications, or draw blood for labs, and she threatened to leave against medical advice. Dr. Anderson had more faith in me than I had. I felt myself tense up as I reviewed her chart.

My pulse quickened when I arrived at her room. I took a deep breath and knocked on the door. There was no answer, so I knocked again, but there was still no answer. I slowly opened the door and entered the dark room. All the lights were off, and the window blind was closed, but some light leaked through. Ms. Flores was asleep in bed, snoring loudly, and I really didn't want to awaken her. She appeared Caucasian, older than her stated age, obese, disheveled, with dirty blonde hair, wearing a hospital gown, oxygen by nasal cannula, and she had an IV line.

"Ms. Flores," I said.

She continued to snore.

"Ms. Flores," I said louder.

She didn't respond.

I moved closer to her bed and called her name again, but she continued to snore. I wanted to call it a day and go home, but what would I tell Dr. Anderson in the morning? That I was afraid to awaken her, but I would be happy to see another patient? I took another deep breath. I touched her shoulder, called her name, and braced myself for a possible assault. She still didn't respond. I gently shook her shoulder and called her name. She quit snoring, but she didn't awaken. I shook her shoulder harder, called her name, and she finally opened her eyes and moved.

"Ms. Flores. Good afternoon," I said. "I'm James. I'm a medical student with the psychiatry consult service."

"Hello," she said. "What time is it?"

"Almost four o'clock."

"Thanks. I'm so tired." She pressed a button to raise the head of her bed up.

"Do you mind if I turn on a light or open the blind?"

"Sure."

"Do you have a preference?"

"I just don't like these bright lights over my bed. Bright lights trigger my migraines, and I get bad migraines that keep me in bed for days."

"That sounds miserable."

"It is."

I partly opened the blind. "How's that?"

"That's fine."

"Do you know why psychiatry was consulted to see you?" I sat in a chair next to her bed.

"My medications aren't right."

"I've reviewed your medication list. Tell me why your medications aren't right."

"I've been flipping out and having bad mood swings. Everyone's been pissing me off, and I almost left the hospital yesterday, even though I could hardly breathe. I've been manicky, and my anxiety's been off the chain."

Ms. Flores proceeded to calmly, appropriately answer my questions, and I was relieved to gather all the pertinent history for her psychiatric evaluation without any drama. At the end of the interview, we discussed potential medication adjustments.

"Can you increase my Xanax?" she said.

"A higher dose of Xanax wouldn't help your mood swings, and it would increase your risk of breathing problems with Percocet," I said.

"Could you add something else to go with my other medicines then?"

"Well, you're already on a polypharmacy regimen with nine medications that affect your brain, including multiple sedating medications. Seroquel, Xanax, trazodone, Percocet, and Flexeril are all sedating medications. I was actually thinking that your regimen needs to be simplified by decreasing or discontinuing medication."

"Seriously?"

"Yes."

"So you're not going to add or increase anything?"

"Well, I can't actually adjust your medications anyway because I'm not a doctor yet. The psychiatry resident and attending will see you in the morning, but they may agree that your regimen needs to be simplified."

Ms. Flores jumped out of bed, turned her back to me, and fiddled with belongings in the shelves next to the head of her bed. Her hospital gown wasn't tied in the back, and she wasn't wearing underwear, so I saw her bare butt.

"I knew they'd send an arrogant motherfucker to see me!" she said angrily.

"I'm sorry—"

"Get the fuck out of here and don't come back!"

"Okay." I left the room. I completed a handwritten note, made a copy, and placed the original in her chart.

The following morning I met the psychiatry team in the doctors' lounge. Everyone was at a table, eating and drinking coffee, except for Laura, who hadn't yet arrived.

"Good morning, James," Dr. Anderson said. "How are you?"

"Okay, except the borderline blew up on me yesterday, and she told me not to come back," I said.

"Really!"

"Yeah."

"Okay. Well, grab a coffee and breakfast and tell us about this borderline."

I got a Starbucks coffee, bacon, scrambled eggs, fresh pineapple, cantaloupe, and strawberries, and I sat at the table.

"Let's wait till Laura gets here for you to present the case," Dr. Anderson said.

"Okay." I started to eat my breakfast.

Laura arrived after a few minutes. "Sorry I'm late."

"It's okay," Dr. Anderson said. "Grab a coffee and breakfast. James has a case to present."

Laura got a coffee and joined us. I formally presented the case, and I described the patient's behavior when she jumped out of bed and showed me her bare buttocks.

"And she cursed me and told me not to come back," I said.

"So she showed you her bare ass, and she cursed you," Dr. Anderson said, smiling. "What exactly did she say? A patient's choice of curse words tells us more about their mental status."

"She said, quote, 'I knew they'd send an arrogant motherfucker to see me.'"

Dr. Anderson laughed heartily, and the others joined him.

I smiled. "I told her I was sorry, but she said, 'Get the fuck out of here and don't come back.'"

They laughed again.

"Did you put all that in your note?" Dr. Anderson said.

"Yes," I said.

"Good."

"I told you she'd be a tough case. Now you just need to stop being so arrogant."

We laughed and finished breakfast. The psychiatry team saw Ms. Flores without me, and I rejoined them. Dr. Anderson told me she apologized for her behavior, and she asked him to tell me that she was sorry. Drs. Rogers and Anderson agreed that her polypharmacy regimen should be simplified, but she politely said she really needed all of her medications. They didn't recommend a medication change, and they advised her to follow up with her psychiatric nurse practitioner at New Horizons.

The psychiatry team met with her family medicine team and nurses. Dr. Anderson said that everyone needed to be on the same page and consistent in dealing with Ms. Flores to prevent her from splitting staff (playing staff against each other), and she should be discharged as soon as she was medically stable. The medical team and nurses said they would be happy to wean her off oxygen as soon as possible to discharge her. Ms. Flores' behavior was much better over the next 24 hours, and she was discharged the following day.

During the third week Tyler and Laura also presented interesting patients they had evaluated, but the patients didn't curse them. Tyler saw a 24-year-old male who had delirium secondary to benzodiazepine withdrawal vs. methamphetamine intoxication vs. schizophrenia. Laura saw a 54-year-old female with syncope, pseudoseizures (psychogenic nonepileptic seizures), and bipolar disorder. Pseudoseizures are seizure-like episodes that occur as somatic manifestations of psychological distress.

On Friday morning I logged into the National Board of Osteopathic Medical Examiners website, and I was happy to see that I PASSED the COMLEX Level 2-Cognitive Evaluation!

At the end of my fourth week, Dr. Anderson told me that Dr. Vaswani had reservations about me potentially being a resident in the program, but he advocated for me. I thanked him for the endorsement and experience. He gave me a great evaluation and said he hoped I would apply to the program.

Endnotes

1. MS Contin: extended-release morphine.
2. q.h.s.: abbreviation for Latin phrase, meaning every night at bedtime.
3. MAR: medication administration record.
4. "C-L": consultation-liaison psychiatry.
5. CK: creatine kinase.

Chapter 14

COMLEX Level 2-Performance Evaluation

On Monday, August 31, I left our apartment at 7 a.m. with a small bag. Lynn and I hugged and kissed and said we loved each other. She told me I'd do great and asked me to drive safely. I got into my Volvo sedan and made a 9.5-hour drive from Brighton to Conshohocken, Pennsylvania (a Philadelphia suburb), for the dreaded COMLEX Level 2-Performance Evaluation. The COMLEX Level 2-PE was a six-hour clinical skills exam. I had to perform history and physicals on 12 "standardized patients" (actors) with different presentations and formulate differential diagnoses and treatment plans. Some of the patients would require osteopathic manipulative treatment for musculoskeletal problems. I was allowed 30 minutes for each encounter, and I had to complete handwritten notes.

I arrived at a Best Western hotel at 4:30 p.m., feeling tired from the long drive and anxious about the next day. The Best Western was 15 minutes from the test facility, and I stayed there because the $64 rate was a third to half the price of closer hotels. I pulled two Fat Tire amber ales out of my bag and put them in a bucket of ice water to chill. I called Lynn to let her know I had reached my destination, and we had a short conversation. She wished me good luck again, and we said we loved each other.

I picked up dinner from a nearby Wendy's, returned to my room, and kicked back on the bed. The spicy chicken sandwich, fries, and beer were especially delicious after a long day on the road. I mindlessly watched TV and finished the second beer, but I had difficulty relaxing. I wished I still had a Xanax prescription. The medication was a lifesaver during my very stressful second year of medical school. I went to sleep at 10 p.m. to get eight hours of sleep, but my sleep was restless. I awakened every one to two hours, looked at the alarm clock, and fell back asleep.

I arrived at the testing center on Tuesday, September 1, at 7:30 a.m. with my stethoscope and white lab coat, which I was required to wear. The facility was in a five-story executive office building. I said hi to several of my classmates when I checked in and registered, and I had orientation with all of the students. I placed my wallet, keys, cell phone, Seiko wristwatch, and lunch in a locker. I had only a chocolate brownie Clif Bar and apple because I didn't want a heavy lunch to make me lethargic in the afternoon. I was only allowed to take my stethoscope and two pens into the exam area. I was perturbed by not being allowed to use my own watch to track time. Clocks were in the exam rooms and throughout the testing center.

Each "patient" had a doorway information sheet that contained their name, age, chief complaint, weight, and vitals.

"You may begin your clinical encounter," a female voice said over speakers.

I rushed to complete six encounters before lunch. My anxiety was intense. My heart raced, and I felt short of breath, hot, and sweaty—I panicked for three hours! I took deep breaths and struggled to stay functional.

"Two minutes remaining," the voice said near the end of each encounter.

I rushed to finish my notes if I hadn't already finished them by the two-minute mark.

"Time is up," the voice said. "Please stop writing. Please rotate to the next station."

I was relieved to finish the sixth station to get a break from the pressure.

"Follow the proctors to the break area," the voice said.

I had 30 minutes to relax and eat my light lunch, but, of course, relaxing was impossible. I didn't feel good about my performance, and I hoped to perform better in the afternoon.

After lunch, I rushed to complete six more encounters. Unfortunately, the afternoon didn't go as I hoped. I walked out of the cool test center shortly after 3 p.m. and went to my car. The thick, hot air was oppressive. I was exhausted, and I felt a sense of despair. I took off my white coat and stethoscope and got into my car. I started the engine, turned the air conditioner on full blast, and called Lynn.

"Hi, babe," I said. "I finished the exam, but I have a bad feeling about it."

"Oh, I'm sure you did fine," she said.

"I don't know. I hope I'm wrong, but I have a bad feeling."

"I'm sure plenty of other students feel that way."

"Maybe. I just hope I don't have to return to Conshofucken, Pennsylvania, to go through that hell again. I have to wait eight to ten weeks to find out if I passed."

"That's ridiculous."

"Tell me about it."

"Well, I'm sure you did fine. Are you heading home now? I miss you."

"Yeah. I should be home around 12:30."

"Please be careful. I love you."

"Okay. I love you too."

I had decided to make the long drive home after the exam because I didn't want to stay another night in Philadelphia and I didn't want to pay for another night in a hotel after paying $1,100 for the exam. Nine and a half hours was a long time to ruminate, and I was glad I had a vacation to look forward to, starting the next day. I drove as fast as I could without the risk of getting a speeding ticket (seven miles an hour over the speed limit), and I listened to rock 'n' roll from my iPod, which was plugged into the premium sound system. When I grew tired of music, I listened to stories from Garrison Keillor's *The News from Lake Wobegon*. I stopped at a Subway to get an Italian BMT sandwich, chips, and a few cookies for dinner, and I ate while

I drove to save time. My eyes grew heavy after six hours, so I stopped at a gas station to get a cup of coffee to carry me through the rest of the trip. I was happy to arrive home in nine hours. I was utterly exhausted. Lynn greeted me with a kiss. I had a bourbon and fell into a very deep sleep.

Chapter 15

Vacation!

A much-deserved vacation started on Wednesday, September 2! I vegetated at home all day long while Lynn worked at the bank. On Thursday I applied to 12 psychiatry residency programs in Kentucky, Tennessee, North Carolina, and Western states. I was happy to be done with my third year of medical school, and I could relax until September 14, when my first emergency medicine rotation was scheduled to start. On Friday after Lynn returned from work, we put packed bags in my car and made a three-hour drive to Cincinnati to stay overnight with our good friends Chris and Jamie Devlin. Chris was my classmate, and he was doing his clinical rotations in Cincinnati. On Saturday we flew to Phoenix, Arizona, and we spent a week in Sedona, exploring the Martian landscape of red sandstone formations. We only had to pay for our flights and rental car because my father didn't plan to use his timeshare for the year.

Our condo was situated on a golf course with a view of some red buttes. We leisurely enjoyed coffee on our patio during the cooler mornings. Temperatures ranged from the low 60s to mid 90s. Sedona's elevation was nearly a mile high, and the climate was arid, so the afternoon heat wasn't nearly as bad as it was in Kentucky.

We explored the area in a Dodge Charger, which was fun to drive, especially through the twists and turns of Oak Creek Canyon northeast of town. We hiked around Bell Rock and Cathedral Rock and slid through an icy creek in Slide Rock State Park. We visited Chapel of the Holy Cross, a Roman Catholic architectural landmark. The chapel is a tall, slender trapezoid of coarse concrete walls and glass ends wedged into buttes and features a 90-foot-tall cross built into the frame that faces the road and valley below. The cross extends deeper into the rock below the floor, and the structure is an impressive sight to behold from the road. The landmarks around Sedona were especially photogenic. I took lots of photos with my Canon professional digital camera, and I photographed Cathedral Rock at sunset when the formation was reflected in Oak Creek.

We enjoyed late, delicious breakfasts at the Coffee Pot Restaurant and delicious dinners and beers at Oak Creek Brewing Co. The Coffee Pot had 101 different omelettes to choose from. Lynn was adventurous enough to try a peanut butter and jelly omelette. She ate the omelette, but she didn't exactly like it. I told her I wasn't surprised, but I commended her for being adventurous.

The only thing that put a small damper on our trip was an email I received in the middle of the week from the University of Colorado's Psychiatry Department. They had received many applications and could not offer me an interview. I had lived in the Colorado Rockies for three years before medical school, and I wanted to return. I enjoyed skiing, snowboarding, mountain biking, hiking, and simply beholding the beauty of God's country. I even had a fun job as a photographer for the *Vail Daily*, but the income was only enough for subsistence living in the expensive resort town. Lynn didn't completely share my interest. She thought Colorado was a beautiful place, but she didn't like cold weather. She was afraid to drive in snowy conditions, and she didn't want to live far away from family. I hadn't received a response from any of the other residency programs I had applied to, so I started to worry about how many more rejections might come. Lynn comforted me, and we still thoroughly enjoyed the rest of our vacation. We were sad when our awesome week came to an end, and we didn't want to return to Brighton.

We returned to our apartment around 5 p.m. on Sunday, and we tried not to think about Monday morning. I had to be at the BMC library at 7 a.m. for morning report, and my ED rotation started at 8 a.m. I was jealous of Lynn not having to be back at work until 9 a.m. We did our best to savor our final few hours of vacation. We kicked back on our bed, watched a romantic comedy, drank a beer, had sex, and fell into a deep sleep.

Chapter 16

Emergency Medicine

My alarm awakened me at 5:50 a.m. I hit the snooze button twice to get 18 precious, extra minutes of sleep, and I dragged myself out of bed. I didn't want to go back to BMC to start my dreaded emergency medicine rotation after returning from our awesome Sedona vacation, but I did want to graduate. I arrived at the medical library at 7 a.m. Dr. Bailey gave a PowerPoint presentation about diabetes management. I was half asleep as usual, and I didn't really care about the topic, even though I knew I'd have to take care of diabetic patients as a psychiatry resident in less than a year.

I was also battling anxiety and pessimism. I feared I had failed the $1,100 COMLEX Level 2-PE, and I really did not want to return to Philadelphia to retake the exam. I also feared I would receive more rejection notices from residency programs. I was only physically present for the morning report because attendance was mandatory and monitored by attendance sheets. Even though I wasn't paying attention to Dr. Bailey's talk, I noticed his idiosyncrasy of shifting his weight from leg to leg, which caused his torso to sway back and forth. The lecture went by exceedingly slowly as I kept checking my watch to see how much time was left. I managed to stay awake, but I had no idea what Dr. Bailey said. After the lecture, I reluctantly went downstairs to start my emergency medicine rotation at 8 a.m. I had plenty of rotations in medicine and surgery under my belt at this point, and I was building confidence, but I still dreaded my ED rotation.

BMC's ED—a haphazard arrangement of rooms—appeared to have been slapped together as an afterthought, and hospital leadership planned to build a properly designed ED. The ED had 20 beds, including six urgent-care beds for patients with lower-priority problems. The rooms were various shapes and sizes, and one larger room had several beds in it, separated by curtains. An enclosed nurses' station was in the center of the ED. The room was long, narrow and had windows facing some patient bays that were separated only by curtains. Patient rooms were on either side of the bays. The "doc box" was a long, narrow room behind the nurses' station. The room had a long, built-in desk with computers.

I went into the doc box and met Brad Penley, M.D. He was medical director of an ED in Louisville, three and a half hours away, and he rarely worked at BMC to cover shifts. Other doctors worked at BMC regularly, but many of them also lived two to three and a half hours away in Lexington or Louisville. Dr. Penley was sitting in front of a computer, reviewing a patient's labs, and he had several paper charts in front of him. He appeared young, handsome, wearing a stethoscope around his neck, and royal blue scrubs. He had the look of a jock who attracted cheerleaders. He wasn't wearing a wedding ring.

"Dr. Penley. Good morning," I said. "I'm James Banks. I'm starting my ED rotation today."

"Good morning, James," he said. "Have a seat."

I sat next to him.

"Are you a fourth-year?"

"Yeah. I'm counting down till graduation now."

"What are you gonna be when you grow up?"

"A psychiatrist."

"Really?"

"Yeah."

"I can't remember the last time I met a student going into psychiatry."

"I think there's only one other student in my class going into it."

"Well, you should see plenty of crazies in the ED." He grinned.

"I'm sure I will."

"Grab a chart." He pointed to a rack on a wall next to the door. The rack had a few charts in it.

I reluctantly got up and pulled a chart out of the rack. At least staying busy would distract me from my worries. The patient was a 78-year-old female with chief complaint of shortness of breath. Her vital signs were: blood pressure 172/109, pulse 112, temperature 97.8, respirations 28, pulse ox 92% on two liters of oxygen by nasal cannula. An EKG had already been done, and it showed no acute ST-segment changes (no obvious heart attack or decreased blood supply to the heart). Q waves appeared to be larger than normal, which could indicate a past heart attack. QRS complexes were tall, which indicated that she had left ventricular hypertrophy.[1] Her medication list included carvedilol, benazepril, atorvastatin, aspirin, nitroglycerin, and Combivent, a combination bronchodilator inhaler.

I went to see the patient, who was fortunate to have one of the few private rooms in the ED. She was reclined in the bed with the head tilted up. She appeared older than her stated age, thin, and frail, with grayish-white hair. She had labored breathing, and her affect was anxious.

"Ms. Ratliff. Hello," I said. "I'm James. I'm a medical student."

"Hi," she said.

"I can see you're having trouble breathing. When did this start?"

She took deep breaths during pauses in her speech. "I woke up earlier than usual this morning, and I just felt like I was smotherin'.... I just couldn't catch my breath. I used my inhaler, but it didn't help.... So I figured I better go to the ER. I've got COPD and heart failure."

"Okay. Have you had this much difficulty breathing before?"

"Yeah. I was in the hospital for a few days a few months ago."

"This hospital?"

"Yeah. I had fluid in my lungs."

"Did you have an echocardiogram[2] while you were in the hospital?"

"I don't know. They ran a bunch of tests, and they took pictures of my heart."

"Okay. Did they tell you what your heart's ejection fraction was?"

"They may have, but I don't recall."

"Okay. Do you have a cardiologist?"

"Yeah. I see Dr. Smith. He's such a nice, handsome doctor.... You're handsome too." She smiled.

I smiled back. "Thank you. Do you smoke?"

"Yeah, but I've cut back."

"Okay. How much have you been smoking?"

"Oh, about a pack a day, but I used to smoke two packs a day."

"When did you start smoking?"

"When I was 16. I didn't smoke so much when I started though."

"Do you use oxygen[3] at home?"

"No."

"Have you had any chest pain?"

"No."

"Have you had a cough?"

"Well, I pretty much always cough some junk up when I get up in the morning.... But my cough has gotten worse."

"What color is the junk you cough up?"

"Greenish yellow."

"Have you noticed any blood in your phlegm?"

"No."

"Have you had any fever or chills?"

"No."

"Have you been taking your medications?"

"I try to, but I don't always remember. My memory's not what it used to be.... And sometimes I get confused and get my pills mixed up.... If I miss my blood pressure pills, my blood pressure goes sky-high.... It was real high when I had fluid in my lungs."

"How high was it?"

"It was around 210 over 120."

"That is real high."

"Yeah. Dr. Smith lectured me about how important it is to take my blood pressure and heart medicines."

"When did you last take your medicines?"

"I think I forgot to take them yesterday."

"Okay. Did you take them this morning?"

"I didn't take any of my pills. I just used my inhaler and called an ambulance right away."

"Do you have anyone at home to help you with your medications?"

"No, honey. It's just me. My husband died nine years ago."

"I'm sorry to hear that."

"Thank you. I still miss him. We were married for 50 years.... But I get along okay now."

"Not many people stay married for 50 years."

"We were high-school sweethearts."

"Do you have any family or friends who could help you out?"

"I could use some help. But my daughter lives in Virginia, and my son's in Ohio."

"What about friends?"

"I don't have any friends either. I'm a homebody."

"Okay. Have you seen Dr. Smith since you were in the hospital?"

"Yeah. I saw him a few weeks ago, and he said everything was alright."

"Have you ever had a heart attack?"

"Well, Dr. Smith told me an EKG showed that I had one in the past.... But I never felt like I had a heart attack."

"Okay. So you had a silent heart attack at some point. Have you ever had a stroke?"

"No."

"Okay. Can I take a listen to your heart and lungs?"

"Sure."

I auscultated her heart and lungs. Her chest was thin, and her heart sounds were faint and dull. I heard a systolic murmur that indicated aortic stenosis, an outflow obstruction. She coughed when I asked her to take deep breaths. She had diminished breath sounds and wheezing due to COPD. I also thought I heard some fine crackles in both lung bases that could indicate pulmonary edema (fluid in the lungs), but I wasn't sure. I examined her abdomen. It was soft and scaphoid (sunken from lack of fat), and my palpation didn't cause any discomfort. I palpated weak radial pulses in both wrists, and I couldn't feel a dorsal pedal pulse in the top of either foot. She didn't have pitting edema in her legs.

"Okay," I said. "Your lungs aren't moving air well. I heard some wheezing and a heart murmur."

"Dr. Smith told me he heard a murmur before," she said.

"Okay. We'll probably get you a breathing treatment, chest x-ray, and some blood work."

"Okay. Thank you." Her breathing was less labored, and she appeared less anxious.

"You're welcome."

I went to the doc box and presented the case to Dr. Penley.

"Okay," he said after I finished. "Have you done an ED rotation before?"

"No," I said.

"Differential diagnosis is important in emergency medicine. What's your differential?"

"COPD exacerbation, heart failure, MI, myocardial ischemia."[4]

"What else?"

"Lung cancer."

"What about a PE?"[5]

"I don't think that's likely. She didn't have any chest pain."

"What kind of chest pain would a PE classically produce?"

"Pleuritic. It would worsen with deep breathing."

"Okay. Why would you include MI and myocardial ischemia in your differential if she had no chest pain?"

"She's 78 years old. Elderly and diabetic patients can have MIs with atypical presentations."

"Okay. What about pneumonia?"

"She hasn't had a fever or blood in her sputum. I think pulmonary edema is more likely than pneumonia."

"I'd still include pneumonia in the differential for this lady though. Thirty percent of elderly patients with pneumonia have no fever, and there's not always blood in the sputum. If she has pulmonary edema, which side of her heart is failing?"

"Left side."

"Yes. Could she also have right heart failure?"

"She doesn't have peripheral edema."

"Okay. What's the most common cause of right heart failure?"

"Left heart failure."

"Yes. How does that happen?"

"Left heart failure can cause pulmonary hypertension, which causes right heart failure."

"Right. Now what do you want to do with this patient, doctor?"

"Well, I'm not a doctor yet."

"You will be soon. When do you graduate?"

"May."

"Okay. So you'll be a doctor in eight months. Now what do you want to do with this patient, doctor?"

I hadn't thought much about actually becoming a doctor soon. The thought was scary! I was too worried about whether

I would have to go back to Philadelphia to retake the COMLEX Level 2-PE, and I wondered if I should apply to 20 residencies, instead of just 12.

I told Dr. Penley my plan for Ms. Ratliff: "Chest x-ray, CMP, CBC, troponin, DuoNeb[6] breathing treatment, and treat her blood pressure."

"Sounds good. We may also get an ABG."[7]

"Okay."

"What would you give her for blood pressure?"

"How about her home meds carvedilol and benazepril?"

"If she's in acute heart failure, would you give her carvedilol?"

"Uh, no. A beta blocker could worsen acute heart failure."

"Right. We'll give her benazepril. And if she has pulmonary edema, we'll give her nitroglycerin and Lasix."

"Okay."

Dr. Penley examined Ms. Ratliff. He also heard crackles in her lung bases and a systolic heart murmur. The chest x-ray confirmed COPD and pulmonary edema, and she was given nitroglycerin and Lasix. Her breathing and pulse ox normalized, but Dr. Smith still accepted her for an observation admission.

I saw a good variety of other patients during my first 12-hour shift in the ED: a 45-year-old male with chest pain, a 36-year-old male with pancreatitis, a 58-year-old female with abdominal pain and pneumonia, a 21-year-old male with fever, a 69-year-old male with syncope, a 76-year-old male with rib pain, a 62-year-old female with knee pain, a 29-year-old female with postpartum hemorrhage after a C-section two weeks earlier, a 76-year-old male with a poison ivy rash on both of his arms, a 65-year-old female with right upper quadrant abdominal pain, right flank pain, and nausea; and an 85-year-old female with constipation and generalized weakness.

Even though I had dreaded my ED rotation, the first day was interesting, and I was distracted from my worries about the COMLEX Level 2-PE and residency applications. I worked seven day and seven night 12-hour shifts with different doctors, and I saw kids and adults with all kinds of problems and injuries. I sutured some lacerations and performed some rectal and vaginal exams, which made me especially glad I had decided to become a psychiatrist. I saw plenty of patients with COPD exacerbations and chest pain, but only one patient actually had an MI. The rotation wasn't nearly as exciting as the ER TV series. Most of the patients did not have true emergencies. Many patients without insurance inappropriately used the ED as their primary care provider. I saw a number of interesting cases, and only two patients died.

Mr. Hurt was a 62-year-old male who presented with dizziness and shortness of breath after he nearly lost consciousness at home. He was on medications for DM and HTN. His BP was stable, pulse was 115, and finger stick blood glucose was mildly elevated. He was in one of the beds in the middle of the ED, and his curtain was open. He was reclined in bed with the head tilted up. He appeared his stated age, obese, diaphoretic (sweaty), well-groomed, balding, with white hair, casually dressed.

"Mr. Hurt. Hello," I said. "I'm James. I'm a medical student."

"Hi, James," he said.

"So you've had dizziness, shortness of breath, and you nearly fainted at home?"

"That's right."

"What happened?"

"I was just mowing the lawn, and I started to feel like I couldn't catch my breath and like I was going to pass out, so I stopped the mower and sat down."

"You were using a push mower?"

"Yeah. I rested for a minute or two, but I still couldn't catch my breath. I started sweating more, and I didn't feel right, so I went to check my blood sugar, but it wasn't too bad. I rested for a little while longer, but I didn't feel any better, and I started to get worried, so I called 911."

"What was your blood sugar?"

"One fifty-two."

"How are you feeling now?"

"Like something's not right, and I can't take a full breath."
He appeared anxious and tachypneic (with rapid breathing).

"Have you had any chest pain?"

"No."

"What about chest pressure or discomfort?"

"No."

"Any numbness or tingling in your arms?"

"No."

"Okay."

I performed a physical exam and went to the doc box to consult with a doctor. An EKG and blood labs were ordered. The EKG only showed sinus tachycardia. The first troponin lab was normal, but six hours later, the second troponin level was abnormally elevated, which indicated damage to the heart muscle. Mr. Hurt was diagnosed with a non-ST-segment elevation myocardial infarction (NSTEMI) because the EKG didn't show ST elevation. The cardiology service accepted him for admission, and he was taken to the cardiac catheterization lab.

Wendy, a 38-year-old female, presented with nausea, vomiting, and diarrhea, and she weighed over 600 pounds! I had never seen a patient so huge before! She required two hospital gowns tied together, and she was too wide for the heavy-duty bed, but she was able to stay on it. She was also malodorous, and she appeared ill and panicky. I was frustrated by the challenges in examining her. I was unable to auscultate her heart or lungs, and I couldn't palpate her pulse. I reminded myself that a human was underneath all the adipose tissue, and I felt sad for her.

Not surprisingly, she had a slew of diagnoses: Pickwickian syndrome (obesity hypoventilation syndrome, a combination of severe, grotesque obesity, low oxygen and high carbon dioxide levels in the blood, somnolence, and debility), HTN, CAD,

A-fib, COPD, obstructive sleep apnea, neurogenic bladder (dysfunctional bladder), GERD, degenerative disc disease with history of cervical fusion surgery, numbness and weakness in upper and lower extremities, major depression, and generalized anxiety. She was diagnosed with urosepsis (sepsis from a urinary tract infection) in the ED and admitted. If she survived the hospitalization, she would live a short, miserable life.

Mr. Fuller, a 55-year-old male, presented with altered mental status. He was in a private room, reclined in bed with the head tilted up, and an older woman was sitting in a chair beside him. He appeared older than his stated age, disheveled, with graying, dark hair, unshaven. He was casually dressed in dirty clothes, and he was tremulous. His pulse was 122, and his BP was 187/118.

"Mr. Fuller. Hello," I said. "I'm James. I'm a medical student."

"Hi, young man," he said. "Where the hell am I?"

"You're in the Brighton Medical Center ER."

"Why am I in an ER? How did I get here?"

"You don't remember how you got here?"

"Would I ask you how I got here if I remembered?" He sounded irritable, and he looked at the woman beside him. "What are you doing here?"

"I brought you here," the woman said.

"Why the hell did you bring me to an ER?" he said.

"Because you weren't acting right."

"What do you mean by that?"

"You were confused. You didn't know where you were, and you were, like, talking to people who weren't really there."

"You're saying I'm crazy? You're the crazy one. I saw the Devil plain as day. I told him I wanted nothing to do with him, but he wouldn't leave. He said he had a special place for me in his kingdom, and that scared the hell out of me."

"That definitely sounds scary," I said. "What's your relation?" I said to the woman.

"I'm his fiancée," she said.

"Okay. What was going on before you noticed he wasn't acting right?"

"He had the shakes since he quit drinking cold turkey a couple of days ago. I tried to tell him not to quit like that. He's had DTs before."

"He's had delirium tremens[8] before?"

"He's had the shakes before, but he's never been like this."

He looked to a corner of the room like he saw something, and he whispered.

"What was he drinking?" I said.

"Jim Beam," she said.

"How much?"

"A fifth[9] every day or two."

"Wow."

"Get thee behind me, Satan!" he said loudly to a corner of the room, suddenly agitated. "I said, get thee behind me, Satan! I want nothing to do with you!" He looked at his girlfriend and me. "I need to get the fuck out of here!"

He bolted up in bed and put his feet on the floor to leave, but he suddenly froze, groaned, became rigid, and his eyes fluttered. He started to fall forward off the bed, but I grabbed his shoulders and pushed him back onto the bed. His eyes rolled up, and he started convulsing. I turned him onto his side, pulled up the bed rails, and ran to grab a doctor.

The doctor ordered an intramuscular Ativan injection because Mr. Fuller didn't yet have an IV line. A nurse quickly administered the injection, and he stopped convulsing after a few minutes, but he remained unconscious for a while. An IV line was placed, and blood was drawn for labs. He received an IV bolus of normal saline with 5% dextrose and IV thiamine, and he was admitted to the ICU.

I can still remember Ms. Osborne's long, messy, brown hair and pale, attractive face like it was yesterday. She was a 23-year-old mother of three, and she presented unconscious after an IV OxyContin overdose. I saw her as soon as she arrived with Brent Johnson, M.D. Her blood drug screen was also positive for Klonopin. She didn't respond to the Narcan antidote, and she had signs of brain damage, including agonal breathing, no response to pain, and fixed, dilated pupils. Dr. Johnson intubated her and connected her to a ventilator, but he told her mother that she might not come out of a coma.

Her mother wailed. "You can't do this, Christine! You hear me! You have to wake up!" She shook her by a shoulder again. "You have to wake up! Wake up!" She stroked her hair and kissed her cheek. "I should have found you sooner. I'm sorry. I love you so much."

Christine Osborne was quickly admitted to the ICU. A week later her mother decided to remove her from the ventilator, and she died.

Mr. Williams, an 18-year-old male, presented with altered mental status and agitation. He was in a private room with his mother. He was standing when I entered the room, and his mother was sitting in a chair. He appeared disheveled, thin, with short, brown hair, unshaven, casually dressed. His mother appeared very worried.

"Mr. Williams. Hello," I said. "I'm James. I'm a medical student."

"Please call me Jack," he said. "Mr. Williams sounds so formal." He laughed. His eye contact was intense, and his affect was elevated.

"Okay, Jack. What brought you to the ER?"

"You'll have to ask my mom. I told her I don't need to be here. This is ridiculous." He paced around the room.

"I've never seen him like this before," his mother said. "He's been talking out of his head, and he's had very strange and scary behavior."

"She thinks I'm crazy, but she's the crazy one. I'm perfectly coherent. I've never been more clear."

"He said his father is Lucifer. He's Jesus, and we poisoned his food with psilocybin."[10]

"Someone definitely put something in my food."

"His father and I are divorced, and he lives with me and my fiancé."

"Do you believe in Jesus Christ?" he said to me.

"Why do you ask me that?" I said.

"Because if you believe in me, you shall be saved."

"You believe you're Jesus Christ?"

He laughed. "Of course not. I believe in Jesus, and I read the Bible. What's wrong with that? Does being a Christian make me crazy?"

"No. But why would you have said you're Jesus, and your father is Lucifer?"

"I didn't mean that literally. Dad is like Lucifer because he doesn't give me more money when I need it. I'm like Jesus because I speak the truth."

His mother said, "His dad gives him a food allowance, but he spends all the money on beer and cigarettes."

"I enjoy beer and cigarettes. What's wrong with that?"

"When did you last have a drink?" I said.

"I had a few beers this morning because Mom was really getting on my nerves."

"Have you used anything else besides beer and cigarettes?"

"I smoke a little weed."

"When did you last use weed?"

"I don't know. A day or two ago."

"How often do you use it?"

"Maybe a few times a week."

"Why were you screaming at the sky?" his mother said.

"I was having a spiritual moment, and I was calling on the Lord."

"Why were you calling on the Lord?"

"To ask for forgiveness and salvation."

"He said he was raped by angels."

"Angels definitely visited me in my sleep."

"He hasn't slept for the past few days."

"I haven't needed sleep. I've had plenty of energy."

"Have angels visited you while you were awake?" I said.

"No. That would be terrifying!" He laughed.

"Have you heard angels' voices?"

"I heard their voices in my sleep, and they were beautiful. Their faces and bodies were beautiful too." He became tearful.

"Have you heard the voice of God or Jesus?"

"No. That would definitely be terrifying!" He laughed. "I pray for God's mercy in Jesus' name."

"Does he answer your prayers?"

"God answers all prayers. He just doesn't always give us the answers we want."

"Why were you standing on an overpass?" his mother said.

"I was just out for a walk. Can I not go for a walk?"

"We've had to call the police three times. He threatened to kill his father and said he was going to die."

"I didn't mean that literally either. You were really pissing me off, and I was angry."

"My fiancé had to lock up his guns."

"Have you had any suicidal or homicidal thoughts?" I said.

"No, but I might become suicidal if I don't get out of here," he said. "Are we done here? Do either of you have any more questions for me? I'm ready to go."

"I need to give you a physical exam if that's okay, and a doctor needs to see you."

"Okay. Whatever."

"Could you have a seat on the bed?"

He sat on the bed, and I examined him. I went to the doc box to consult with Timothy May, D.O., and we returned to see the patient together. Dr. May was middle-aged, tall, overweight, balding, disheveled, with a thick beard. He wore wrinkled, jade scrubs, and he had a nasty habit of dipping tobacco while he worked. He spit tobacco juice into a plastic soda bottle at his desk. Jack wasn't happy when Dr. May informed him that he couldn't leave because he needed to be admitted to a psychiatric hospital.

"You're saying I have to go to a crazy house!" Jack said. "This is ridiculous! I'm not crazy! I've never been more clear!"

"Whenever we have a concern for safety, we err on the side of caution," Dr. May said. "We just want to make sure you and your family stay safe."

"Well, I'm sorry, but I'm not going to a loony bin. Okay, Mom. I have officially been evaluated. Can we go home now?"

"You need help, Jack," his mother said with tears in her eyes.

He yelled, "What I need is to get the fuck out of here! I'm definitely suicidal now!" He jumped off the bed, kicked the red biohazard waste can, and swiped a plastic jar of tongue depressors off the sink counter. The jar hit the floor, and the tongue depressors spilled all over the floor.

"You need to sit back down," Dr. May said firmly. "We don't tolerate violent behavior in the Emergency Department."

"I don't want to sit down." He made a quick move like he was going to bolt for the door, which was behind Dr. May and me.

We flinched, and he laughed.

"Please sit down," Dr. May said.

He stared at us intensely, smiled, and laughed again.

"Jack, please sit down," his mother said.

"No," he said. "I refuse to sit down, and I refuse to be locked up with a bunch of crazy people. I'm not crazy."

"I can give you some good medicine to help you calm down," Dr. May said.

"How about a beer instead?"

"Sorry. I can't order you a beer."

"What do you want to give me then?"

"A shot of Haldol, Ativan, and Benadryl."

"A shot!"

"It works quicker than pills."

"And you think I need three medications!"

"It's a combination that works very well for calming agitated patients."

"Whatever. Jesus Christ is my savior!" He became tearful again. "Have you been saved?"

"You'll take the shot then?"

"Whatever." He looked up to the ceiling. "I call upon you Lord to deliver me from this hell!" He laughed.

We left the room and shut the door.

He yelled, "Jesus Christ is my savior! I am Jesus! Believe in me, and you shall not perish but have everlasting life!"

A nurse had two injections ready in a few minutes. Haldol and Ativan were in one syringe, and Benadryl was in the other. Dr. May and I accompanied her to Jack's room. He accepted the injections without incident, and he was asleep 30 minutes later. A psychiatrist at Luray Behavioral Health Center accepted him for admission, but he had to wait until the next day for a bed to become available. He was fortunate that he didn't have to wait several days for a bed as psych patients often did.

Mr. Yates, a 30-year-old male, presented with shortness of breath and ventricular tachycardia, a type of arrhythmia that can be life-threatening. I saw him as soon as he arrived with Charles Potter, D.O. Dr. Potter was a young, fit, countryman with a thick beard, and he wore jade scrubs. He liked to hunt and fish. He didn't dip tobacco while he worked, but one evening he opened his duffle bag to show another ED doc a Judge revolver he recently purchased. The Judge is a five-round pistol that can shoot .45 Colt and .410 shotgun shells.

Mr. Yates had tetralogy of Fallot, a rare set of four congenital heart defects: ventricular septal defect (hole in the septum between right and left ventricles), pulmonary valve stenosis (constriction of the valve), dextroposition of the aorta (right-shifted aorta overrides the ventricular septum and receives deoxygenated blood from the right ventricle and oxygenated blood from the left ventricle), and right ventricular hypertrophy (reactive enlargement of the right ventricle). Mr. Yates had open-heart surgery to repair the defects when he was an infant.

Two paramedics rushed him into the ED on a gurney, and his father was with him. The patient had messy, blond hair, and he appeared ill, pale, tachypneic, wearing oxygen by nasal cannula. His father appeared old enough to be his grandfather. He was thin, disheveled, balding, with gray hair, wearing tattered clothes.

The patient was placed on a bed in a curtained bay that was visible from the nurses' station. A nurse connected him to hospital oxygen. He removed his shirt, and she placed sensors on his chest for vitals monitoring. He had a midline scar on his chest from heart surgery. The monitor alarm dinged due to ventricular tachycardia. The nurse placed an IV in his left forearm.

"I love you, Dad," Mr. Yates said.

"I love you too, son," his father said.

"He's going into V-fib,"[11] Dr. Potter said.

Mr. Yates lost consciousness.

Dr. Potter palpated his wrist and neck. "He has no pulse. Call a code blue. Let's start CPR."

I started hard and fast chest compressions (100 per minute). The nurse called in the code, and another person announced the code over the hospital intercom. The nurse grabbed the crash cart and turned on the defibrillator. While I continued compressions, she quickly shaved the right upper chest and left lower chest, and placed an adhesive defibrillator pad over each area. Another nurse and a respiratory therapist arrived to assist. The nurse started taking notes to record the code. The respiratory therapist removed the nasal cannula from the nose, grabbed a bag valve mask, and connected it to oxygen. He placed the mask over the nose and mouth and squeezed the bag twice to give breaths.

"Charge the defibrillator to 200 joules," Dr. Potter said.

"Okay. Charging to 200 joules." The bedside nurse set the energy level and charged the defibrillator to deliver a shock.

"Stop compressions," Dr. Potter said.

I stopped chest compressions, and Dr. Potter palpated a wrist.

"Let's give him a shock," he said.

"Okay. Clear the patient. Clear the oxygen," the bedside nurse said.

The respiratory therapist removed the mask from the face.

"Everyone's clear. Ready to shock." The bedside nurse pressed the shock button, and the chest jolted. "Shock delivered."

The monitor alarm continued to ding.

"He's still in V-fib." Dr. Potter palpated a wrist. "Resume CPR."

The respiratory therapist and I switched roles, and we gave five cycles of CPR. Each cycle consisted of 30 compressions and two breaths.

"Stop compressions," Dr. Potter said.

The respiratory therapist stopped chest compressions, and Dr. Potter palpated a wrist.

"Let's give him another shock at 300 joules," he said.

"Okay. Charging to 300 joules," the bedside nurse said. "Everyone's clear. Oxygen is clear. Ready to shock." She pressed the shock button, and the chest jolted. "Shock delivered."

The monitor alarm continued to ding.

Dr. Potter palpated a wrist. "Resume CPR and give him one milligram of epinephrine."

I resumed chest compressions, and the respiratory therapist resumed ventilation. The bedside nurse injected epinephrine into his IV. We gave another five cycles of CPR.

"Stop compressions," Dr. Potter said.

I stopped chest compressions, and Dr. Potter palpated a wrist.

"He now has pulseless electrical activity," he said. "Give him another milligram of epinephrine and resume CPR." He didn't order another shock because pulseless electrical activity (PEA) isn't a shockable rhythm.

The bedside nurse gave another dose of epinephrine, and we resumed CPR. The nurse continued to give epinephrine after each five cycles of CPR, but PEA persisted. Other staff took turns giving chest compressions, which was tiring. The PEA rate slowed, and the bedside nurse gave three doses of atropine, which was the recommended maximum. Dr. Potter ran the code for over an hour, even though the return of spontaneous circulation was very unlikely after 30 minutes of CPR. Mr. Yates died in the middle of the night.

His father lived an hour away, and he couldn't afford to stay in a hotel in Brighton. Dr. Potter asked a hospital administrator if the father could stay in a private room for the rest of the night, but the request was denied, even though plenty of beds were available. Dr. Potter called the Holiday Inn Express and paid for a room.

I felt a strong mix of emotions. I felt very sad for the father. I was incensed that the administrator was so heartless. And I was moved by Dr. Potter's compassion. Dr. Potter looked exhausted and disheartened. But he had to continue with the rest of his shift, and moving on to the next patient was not easy.

By the end of my rotation, I had happily accepted a few psychiatry residency interview offers, and I had received no more rejections. I worked with Dr. Potter the most during my rotation, so he completed my evaluation. I thanked him for the experience.

Endnotes

1. Left ventricular hypertrophy (LVH) is enlargement of the left chamber of the heart that pumps blood into the aorta, the main artery. LVH is typically caused by uncontrolled hypertension. The ventricle enlarges because the muscle has to squeeze blood into the aorta against greater resistance.

2. Echocardiogram: ultrasound imaging that is used to examine the structures and functioning of the heart.

3. Oxygen is one of only three treatments that have been shown to decrease morbidity and mortality associated with COPD. The other two treatments are smoking cessation and lung volume reduction surgery in selected patients with emphysema.

4. Myocardial ischemia: inadequate circulation of blood to the myocardium (heart muscle).

5. PE: pulmonary embolism: obstruction of a pulmonary artery by a blood clot.

6. DuoNeb is a combination bronchodilator.

7. ABG: arterial blood gas.

8. "DTs": delirium tremens (severe alcohol withdrawal) is characterized by tremulousness, disorientation, confusion, agitation, hallucinations, seizures, fever, sweating, tachycardia, and hypertension. Up to 15% of treated cases and 35% of untreated cases are fatal.

9. Prior to 1980 liquor and wine were in bottles that were 1/5 of a gallon (757 mL), which is very close to today's 750-mL bottle (16.9 servings of alcohol).

10. Psilocybin: hallucinogenic mushrooms.

11. Ventricular fibrillation (V-fib) is the most serious type of arrhythmia. The ventricles quiver instead of contracting to pump blood. It is the most frequent cause of sudden cardiac death.

Chapter 17

Cardiology

I didn't exactly look forward to my cardiology rotation with Rajesh Singh, M.D., in October, but I was required to complete a medicine subspecialty rotation. Dr. Singh was an FMG with a medical degree from Pakistan. He had completed a three-year internal medicine residency, a three-year cardiology fellowship, and a one-year interventional cardiology fellowship in the U.S.

BMC's shiny Heart Center clinic was on the first floor of the hospital. I arrived at the clinic on Friday at 8 a.m., and I met Dr. Singh in the break room. He was standing, sipping a cup of coffee, chatting with a couple of nurses and his colleague George Smith, M.D. Dr. Singh appeared middle-aged, short, handsome, wearing jade scrubs and a white lab coat with a stethoscope in a pocket. Dr. Smith was dressed the same, and he appeared older and handsome.

"I like your hair," Dr. Smith said to the young, cute nurse. "Did you do something different with it?" He smiled charismatically.

"Thanks, Dr. Smith, but I'm happily married," she said.

"Well, that's great. Can I not simply pay you a compliment?"

"You're divorced from your third wife, and you're on the prowl."

"I just said your hair looks nice."

"Why don't you look for a single woman who's closer to your age?"

"Thanks for the dating advice."

"You're welcome."

"Dr. Singh. Good morning," I said. "I'm James Banks."

"Welcome, James," Dr. Singh said. "Would you like a cup of coffee?"

"No thanks. I've had a cup already."

"Good morning, James," Dr. Smith said. "You're tall. Did you play basketball in school?"

"No. I was actually better at tennis."

"I play tennis," Dr. Smith said. "What specialty have you chosen?"

"Psychiatry."

"Really?"

"Yeah."

"Interesting. Are you a little off?" He smiled.

"Maybe." I smiled back.

"Are you ready to see some patients?" Dr. Singh said.

"Sure."

"I have some patients upstairs. You can go see them, and I'll join you in a little while. I have some echocardiograms to read. Make a copy of my list."

"Okay."

I made a copy of the list and went upstairs to see the six patients: a 78-year-old female and 68-year-old male who had pacers placed, a 70-year-old male with peripheral vascular disease, a 62-year-old male with unstable angina (chest pain), a 67-year-old male with chest pain and altered level of consciousness, and Ms. Slone, a 53-year-old train wreck.

Ms. Slone had CHF, CAD with history of coronary artery bypass graft (CABG) of two arteries, COPD, uncontrolled DM, HTN, HLD, and chronic kidney disease (CKD). She was admitted to the hospitalist service, and cardiology was consulted. She was wearing oxygen by nasal cannula, and she was reclined in bed with the head tilted up, watching TV. She appeared obese, older than her stated age.

"Ms. Slone. Good morning," I said. "I'm James. I'm a medical student working with Dr. Singh."

"Good morning," she said. "Who's Dr. Singh?"

"He's a cardiologist who has been consulted to see you."

"Okay."

"How are you feeling?"

"Much better now."

"Good. What brought you to the hospital?"

"I was smotherin'."

"Were you taking all your medications before you started smothering?"

"I was out of them for a while."

"Why was that?"

"I kept forgetting to go to the pharmacy to get my refills."

"How long were you off your medications?"

"A week or two."

"With your heart condition and all your other medical conditions, it's very important to stay on your medications."

"I know. I'm a bad patient. I'll try to do better."

"You probably wouldn't be in the hospital if you hadn't run out of your medications. You had difficulty breathing because your heart failure worsened and caused fluid to back up in your lungs."

"I know."

"You also have COPD. Are you a smoker?"

"Yeah, but I've cut back."

"Okay. How much are you smoking now?"

"Seven to eight cigarettes a day."

"How much were you smoking before?"

"A pack a day."

"That's good that you've cut back, but it would be better for you to quit altogether. Smoking increases your risk of having a heart attack or stroke, especially with all of your other risk factors. You've had open-heart surgery, and you have poorly controlled diabetes, high blood pressure, and high cholesterol. If you keep smoking and don't take your medications consistently, it's only a matter of time till you have a stroke or heart attack."

"I know. I'll do better."

"Okay. Let me take a listen to you."

I auscultated her heart and lungs. Her heart sounds were faint and dull, and her lung sounds were diminished due to COPD. I palpated a weak radial pulse, and I couldn't feel a dorsal pedal pulse in the top of either foot. She had pitting leg edema, which indicated right heart failure.

"Dr. Singh will see you soon," I said.

"Okay. Thank you," she said.

"You're welcome."

I went to the doctors' room and sat in front of a computer. Dr. Singh wasn't there yet, but hospitalist Dr. Akers was a few seats away with some charts next to him.

"Good morning, Dr. Akers," I said.

"Hello there. How are you?" he said.

"Alright. I just started cardiology with Dr. Singh. How are you?"

"Oh, you know, just stamping out disease and saving lives."

"Of course. I just saw a train wreck who really needs some stamping. She was admitted for a CHF exacerbation after being off her medications for a week or two because she kept forgetting to go to the pharmacy to get refills."

"Noncompliant train wrecks ensure our job security."

"Ha ha! Have you flown your plane recently?"

"I flew to Charleston last month to go to the beach."

"Cool."

"Yeah. It was a nice trip. I got a little sunburned and drank too many margaritas."

"Uh-oh."

"It's okay. I didn't get into any trouble."

"Good. Well, I'll let you get back to it. I just wanted to say hi."

"Okay. Have a good day."

"Thanks. You too."

I spent some more time reviewing charts and making my own notes about the cases. I checked my email and read a few news stories. Dr. Singh arrived, and I presented the cases to him.

"What are we going to do for Ms. Slone?" he said.

"Tell her to be compliant with her medications or she's going to die," I said.

Dr. Singh laughed. "That's true."

"I stressed the importance of medication compliance."

"Good."

We saw the patients together, and I was happy to return home in the early afternoon on Friday.

On Monday morning I rounded on hospitalized patients. Ms. Varney was 94 years old. She was admitted for an NSTEMI, CHF, diabetic ketoacidosis (DKA), and acute renal failure (ARF). "She's just old," I thought, remembering Dr. Coleman. She was asleep in bed when I entered the room. She was wearing oxygen by nasal cannula, and she appeared frail but younger than her stated age.

"Ms. Varney," I said.

She didn't move.

"Ms. Varney," I said louder.

She didn't respond, so I gently touched her shoulder, and she awakened.

"Good morning," I said. "I'm James. I'm a medical student working with Dr. Singh."

"What?" she said.

"I'm James," I said louder. "I'm a medical student working with Dr. Singh."

"Okay. Good morning, young man."

"How are you doing?"

"What?"

"How are you doing?" I said louder.

"Oh, alright, I guess, considering I'm in the hospital."

"How did you end up in the hospital?" I said loudly.

"I had trouble breathing, and they told me I had a heart attack."

"You did have a heart attack, and you've also had heart failure, kidney failure, and diabetic ketoacidosis."

"Well, I am 94 years old."

"That's true." I smiled. "I guess you're blessed with longevity genes. Were you taking your medications before you were hospitalized?"

"Yes, but sometimes I get confused. My daughter helps me with my medicines."

"Does your daughter live with you?"

"Yes. Can I go home today? I hate hospitals."

"Well, we want to make sure you're well enough to go home. Let me take a listen to you."

"Okay."

I auscultated her heart and lungs, palpated her radial and pedal pulses, and left the room. Dr. Singh convinced her to stay in the hospital a little longer.

During the afternoon I saw a couple of patients in the clinic: a 68-year-old male with CAD, HTN, and an automatic implantable cardioverter defibrillator (AICD); and a 63-year-old male with CAD, A-fib, and severe mitral regurgitation.[1] Dr. Singh gave me a caliper to measure EKG wave intervals. I wasn't confident in reading EKGs, but it was easy to see the A-fib. The mitral regurgitation had been diagnosed with an echocardiogram, and I could easily hear a blowing holosystolic murmur when I auscultated the patient's heart. He was on atorvastatin to reduce cholesterol, aspirin to reduce stroke risk, and metoprolol for heart rate control. He was referred to a cardiac surgeon for repair of his badly leaking valve.

I followed Ms. Varney the next day, and I saw a patient in the ICU. The ICU had a nurses' station in the middle of a large room, and patient rooms with sliding glass doors surrounded the station. I felt uncomfortable in the ICU. Patients teetered on the brink of death. Some of the patients were unconscious on ventilators, and they were connected to lots of lines, wires, and bags of medications and fluids.

As I was going to the ICU, I passed an emotional scene in the hall just outside the entrance. A middle-aged, black male intensivist was having a very difficult conversation with a patient's three distraught family members.

"There must be something else you can do!" a woman said while crying.

"I'm very sorry," the doctor said with a thick, exotic accent. "He has multisystem organ failure, and he hasn't responded to treatment. The damage to his organs has been too severe."

"Well, we don't want him unplugged," a man said angrily. "Maybe he just needs some more time to get better."

"I'm very sorry, but we have done all we can do," the doctor said.

I entered the ICU, thinking about how hard it would be to be an intensivist. I went to the nurses' station to review the chart for Mr. Moore. He was 46 years old, and he was on postoperative day one (day after surgery), recovering from a CABG of four arteries after he had an MI. His vitals were stable, and weight was normal. He was on oxygen by mask, IV norepinephrine to keep his blood pressure up, and aspirin to reduce the risk of vein graft occlusion. I entered his room. He was asleep in bed with the head tilted up. He appeared his stated age, and his face was clean-shaven.

"Mr. Moore," I said.

He awakened.

"Mr. Moore, good morning. I'm James. I'm a medical student working with your cardiologist Dr. Singh."

"Hello," he said through the mask, which muffled his voice.

"How are you feeling?"

"Like I've been run over by a truck."

"Well, you did have your chest cracked open."

"I sure did, and God has blessed me with another day."

"You had a heart attack before your surgery."

"Yeah. I was at work, but I wasn't doing anything strenuous. My arms suddenly became numb. I was short of breath, and I felt an intense pressure in my chest, like an elephant was on top of me. I knew I was having a heart attack, so I called 911."

"What do you do for work?"

"I manage the House of Mercy store."

"Did you know you had heart disease?"

"No. I haven't seen a doctor in years, besides my psychiatrist."

"What do you see a psychiatrist for?"

"Depression, anxiety, insomnia. I started seeing Dr. Damron a few years ago when I started my recovery."

"What are you in recovery from?"

"Alcohol."

"Congratulations."

"Thank you. I give the credit to God. I wouldn't have been able to stay in recovery without him. My life was out of control before. My wife divorced me after my third DUI, and I was homeless before the House of Mercy took me in."

"You still live at the House of Mercy?"

"Yes."

"Okay. Are you a smoker?"

"No. Apparently, I just have terrible cholesterol."

"Well, it's nice to see a patient in recovery. Let me take a listen to you."

"Okay."

I auscultated his heart and lungs, palpated his radial and pedal pulses, and examined his chest. He had a bandage over his breastbone and wound drains. I left the room. Dr. Singh met me at the nurses' station, and I presented the case to him.

"Okay," he said. "He's on norepinephrine and aspirin. What other medications should we give him?"

"A statin,[2] a beta blocker, and an ACE inhibitor, or ARB,"[3] I said. "But should antihypertensives be held until he's off norepinephrine?"

"Yes. And what if his cholesterol were normal? Should he still start a statin?"

"My guess is yes since you ask the question."

"Right."

During the afternoon I saw two patients in the clinic: a 55-year-old female with DM who was following up for a normal stress test result, and a 79-year-old male with hypertrophic obstructive cardiomyopathy (HOCM). The elderly man was fortunate to still be alive. His father had died of sudden cardiac death at age 28, so the father probably had a severe form of HOCM. The rare condition is usually caused by inherited gene mutations that cause the heart muscle to grow abnormally thick with disorganized muscle fibers. The severity of HOCM is highly variable. Most patients are asymptomatic throughout life, but some have severe symptoms, and young males have a greater risk of sudden cardiac death.

Over the next few days, I continued to follow Ms. Varney and Mr. Moore, and I saw other hospitalized patients with CAD, CHF, and an NSTEMI. I observed Dr. Singh catheterize the patient with the NSTEMI, and he placed two coronary stents.

"Okay, James," he said as he was finishing the procedure. "What should her medication regimen include?"

"Aspirin, Plavix,[4] a statin, beta blocker, and an ACE inhibitor or ARB."

"Yes."

Ms. Varney was discharged on Thursday, and Mr. Moore was discharged on Friday.

During my second week I saw Elsie Hackney in the clinic as a nurse was taking her to an exam room. She was one of our upstairs neighbors, and she was pleasant. She was older, frail, pale, with curly, white hair. She knew I was a medical student, so she told me about her medical problems as my friends and family did. She had severe CHF (ejection fraction 25%) and COPD. She occasionally smoked a cigarette, and I once gently scolded her when I caught her. She was divorced and estranged from her daughter, her only child, so she was lonely. A nephew occasionally visited her.

"Hi, Elsie," I said.

"Hi, James," she said. "Are you learning lots here?"

"Trying to. How are you?"

"I've been better. I'm here to see Dr. Smith. I had a real scare last week. My defibrillator woke me up in the middle of the night and shocked me a few times, so I went to the ER."

"I'm sorry to hear that."

"I'm glad I have Dr. Smith."

"I'm glad you do too. I hope you don't get shocked again anytime soon."

"Me too. Well, I'll see you around."

"Okay. Don't hesitate to knock on our door if you need anything."

"Thank you. It is comforting to know I have a student doctor living below me."

During my second week I also saw an obese 70-year-old male who had a rocky recovery after a CABG. Prior to surgery he was on Plavix for a coronary stent placed at age 55. The medication was held after surgery to decrease bleeding risk, and he had a stroke after he was transferred from the ICU to a step-down room. Fortunately, the stroke only caused some coordination difficulty with his left hand. But he had to be transferred back to the ICU because he required norepinephrine to keep his blood pressure up and he couldn't be weaned off oxygen due to pulmonary edema. Then on Friday, postoperative day four, he developed A-fib, and he was given two doses of amiodarone for cardioversion (restoration of normal heart rhythm). When I returned to the hospital on Monday, his blood pressure was stable without norepinephrine, and he was back on metoprolol and Plavix. He was able to walk without oxygen, so he was discharged.

By my third week I had happily accepted more psychiatry residency interview offers and declined offers from the University of Arizona, Mayo Clinic, and Oregon Health Sciences University. I received the UA offer after I booked a multi-destination trip for my Western interview tour, which included an interview with Southern Arizona University. I didn't want to live in Rochester, Minnesota, and Oregon was so far away from family. On Thursday afternoon I drove three and a half hours to Louisville to stay overnight for a Friday interview with the University of Louisville program. The psychiatry department paid for my room at the downtown Marriott, which was greatly appreciated! The hotel was within walking distance of the UofL Hospital.

My interview day was a busy, exciting experience. The air was cool, and trees were turning yellow, orange, and red. I wore a tie and my gray pinstripe wool suit. A continental breakfast was provided when I arrived at the Department of Psychiatry at 8 a.m. The residency coordinator and residents were very welcoming, and I met other well-dressed residency candidates from around the country, including Dr. Bailey's son Andy, who was attending the Touro University D.O. school in California. Andy was wearing a suit and tie, and he was handsome and clean-shaven, but his dark hair was long and disheveled. He was also quiet.

I individually interviewed with the residency program director, two faculty members, and the chair of the department. The chair had a large corner office on an upper level of the medical school that had large windows and great views of downtown Louisville. A few residents gave the candidates a tour of UofL's nice facilities, told us about the program and call responsibilities, and answered our questions.

I asked about moonlighting opportunities as I planned to do during all of my interviews. The morning was a blur. At 12 p.m. we had lunch with residents at a nearby Panera Bread restaurant, compliments of the psychiatry department. We had casual conversation and asked more questions. The residents appeared well-rested, happy, and they had good work-life balance, which were good signs. I figured that the residents were also assessing us.

I drove home after lunch and arrived half an hour before Lynn. When she returned home from work, I happily told her about my day. On Sunday afternoon I drove to Hansen, Tennessee, to stay overnight for a Monday interview with the University of Northeast Tennessee psychiatry residency. The psychiatry department also paid for my room at the Holiday Inn Express, which was greatly appreciated!

My UNT interview schedule was like the UofL schedule, but I was the only candidate interviewing for the day. Program director Dr. Vaswani was weird, unlike assistant program director Dr. Anderson, who was normal. Most of the residents were also from India, whereas most of the UofL residents were Americans. An Indian and American resident gave me a tour of Hansen's psychiatric hospital and the Veterans Affairs clinic waiting room, but they didn't show me the rest of the clinic or the VA psychiatric hospital, which was curious because the program was based at the VA and residents did most of their rotations there. Hansen's psychiatric hospital and the VA clinic were run-down, dim, and depressing. I had lunch with a few residents at the Main Street Grill, compliments of the psychiatry department. They didn't appear happy, and one of them told me I asked a lot of questions. These were not good signs, which was disappointing because Lynn and I wanted to move back to Hansen.

During the last week of my cardiology rotation—which was eight weeks after I took the COMLEX Level 2-PE—I started anxiously logging into the National Board of Osteopathic Medical Examiners (NBOME) website every day to see if my exam result was available. My pulse quickened every time I logged in.

I saw a couple of interesting cases in the hospital. A 33-year-old morbidly obese male had presented to the ED with chest pain, dizziness, diaphoresis, and he had dextrocardia with situs inversus, obstructive sleep apnea, and depression. Dextrocardia with situs inversus is a rare condition characterized by abnormal positioning of the heart in the right side of the chest and mirror-image reversal of the organs in the chest and abdomen. EKG and serial troponins were negative for MI. The ED doc advised him that he probably had a panic attack, and he was admitted for observation. Dr. Singh discharged him the next day and advised him to follow up in the clinic.

Mr. Collins was 18 years old, and he was admitted for infective endocarditis, a rare disease characterized by inflammation of the innermost lining of the heart and its valves. He contracted a staphylococcal blood infection and hepatitis C from IV heroin use. He was sitting up in bed, watching TV, connected to IV antibiotics. He appeared older than his stated age and underweight with sunken cheeks. He was unshaven, with disheveled, dark hair, wearing a hospital gown.

"Mr. Collins. Good morning," I said. "I'm James. I'm a medical student working with Dr. Singh, a cardiologist who's been consulted to see you."

"Good morning," he said.

"How are you feeling?"

"A lot better than I was now that the antibiotics are kicking in."

"You had a staph infection in your blood from IV heroin use, and the infection went to your heart."

"That's what the doc told me. I just started feeling really sick a few days ago. I was hot and cold. I soaked my sheets with sweat at night, and I had muscle aches. Then I started getting these red spots all over, so I came to the ER." He showed me his arms.

"Those are petechiae."

"And I have these little red bumps on the ends of my fingers, and they hurt."

"Those are Osler's nodes, another sign of a heart infection." I had done some quick reading about infective endocarditis prior to seeing him.

"I guess this is my wake-up call. I need to stay off the dope for good this time. I've been to detox a few times, but I just couldn't stay clean after I got out. I think I need to find me a box doc."

"What's a box doc?"

"A Suboxone doctor."

"Okay."

"Can you give me something for cravings? They're really intense."

"You're on an opioid withdrawal protocol with clonidine."

"That doesn't do anything. It's like taking a Tic Tac."

"You're only 18 years old. How long have you been using heroin?"

"I had my first taste when I was 12."

"Wow!"

"Yeah. I started snorting hillbilly heroin when I was 11, then I started shooting it. But I couldn't get enough pills, so I switched to real heroin."

"How were you getting OxyContin when you were 11 years old?"

"My uncle had the Oxys."

"How did you get the pills from him?"

"He gave them to me."

"Why did he give them to you?"

"'Cause he's a piece of shit, I guess. My mom overdosed when I was 10, and I went to live with him."

"That's really sad."

"Yeah. I guess my family is cursed."

"What about your father?"

"I never met him."

"I'm sorry to hear that."

"It's okay. He's just a sperm donor."

"Okay. Is your uncle your mother's brother?"

"Yeah. I had a really hard time after Mom died. I got started on the junk when I was having a really bad day, and my uncle gave me an Oxy and told me it would help me feel better. He had a prescription, but he didn't take the pills like he was supposed to. He crushed 'em and snorted lines from the coffee table in the living room of his crappy trailer. Then he started shooting up, and I did it with him. He kept running out of pills early, and his doc cut him off. He couldn't find another pill mill, and he couldn't get enough pills off the street, so he got heroin, and he got into the dope business."

"Are you still living with him?"

"No. He went to prison for slinging dope. I've got my own place now."

"Are you still in school?"

"No. I dropped out in seventh grade. I need to get my GED."

"What are you doing now?"

"I've been slinging dope, but I can't keep doing that, or I'll end up in prison like my uncle."

"Well, I hope this is your wake-up call so you can stay off the dope for good this time. You still have your life ahead of you, but you need to change course. Have you been to NA meetings before?"

"I tried a few meetings, but I don't care to hear other people's using stories. That just makes me want to use. And religion doesn't work for me."

"Well, Suboxone certainly sounds better than IV heroin. You also have hepatitis C."

"Yeah. Do you know where I can get treated for that?"

"You'd have to talk to your primary care doctor about that."

"I don't have a doctor."

"Well, you should see one after you get out of here. I'm sure you'll get a referral. Let me take a listen to your heart."

I auscultated his heart and heard a systolic murmur, which meant that he probably had tricuspid valve regurgitation[5] caused by staph vegetations on the valve. Dr. Singh reviewed his echocardiogram and advised him to follow up in the clinic.

On Friday I thanked Dr. Singh for the experience, and he gave me a high B evaluation.

Endnotes

1. Mitral regurgitation is a condition in which the mitral valve doesn't close completely, causing blood to leak back into the left atrium when the left ventricle contracts to pump blood into the aorta.

2. Statins are cholesterol-reducing medications.

3. Angiotensin converting enzyme inhibitors (ACEIs) and angiotensin receptor blockers (ARBs) are antihypertensive medications.

4. Plavix is an antiplatelet medication.

5. Tricuspid valve regurgitation is a condition in which the tricuspid valve doesn't close completely, causing blood to leak back into the right atrium when the right ventricle contracts to pump blood into the pulmonary artery.

Chapter 18

A Mixed Bag

I started my second boring pediatric rotation with Dr. Patel at the beginning of November as the days were turning colder, leaves were falling, and people stopped mowing their lawns. On Friday of my first week, I returned home about half an hour before Lynn. I sat in front of our iMac on the small desk in our living room, and my pulse quickened. I logged into the NBOME website. A surge of adrenaline shot through my chest and took my breath away, then my heart sank. I had FAILED the COMLEX Level 2-PE as I feared. I passed the Biomedical/Biomechanical Domain, but my data gathering, OMT, and note skills "needed improvement." I wasn't "proficient" with any of the skills. I failed the Humanistic Domain, which meant that my people skills sucked. My performance was "poor" with doctor-patient communication, interpersonal skills, and professionalism. I checked dates to retake the exam, poured myself a bourbon, sank into the couch, and turned on the TV.

Lynn entered the apartment and hung up her keys and purse.

"Hey, babe," she said. "Thank goodness it's Friday!"

"Yeah. I failed the COMLEX," I said.

"That's not funny."

"I'm not kidding, unfortunately."

"Seriously?"

"I'm afraid so."

"Oh, honey, I'm so sorry." She took off her shoes and sat beside me.

"Me too. Now I have to pay another eleven hundred dollars plus travel expenses to go back to Conshofucken, Pennsylvania, to retake that damn exam."

"I'm so sorry."

"This won't look good on my residency applications either. I can take the exam again on December 17, which will give me less than six weeks to study. Then I'll have to wait another eight to ten weeks for the result."

"That's ridiculous that you have to wait that long to get your result."

"Yeah, but I should get the result about a month before Match Day.[1] I should have plenty of time to study since I'm on pediatrics now, and I only have to do 14 ED shifts next month."

"Good. You're going to study hard and pass it this time. I believe in you."

"Thanks, babe. I'm going to study my ass off."

"I love you, James." She hugged and kissed me.

"I love you too."

After I was hit with the bad news, I was glad I was on my second boring pediatric rotation. I logged back into the NBOME website and paid another $1,100 to schedule my exam. I purchased a used copy of First Aid for the USMLE Step 2 CS (M.D. clinical skills exam) to study for the COMLEX Level 2-PE. There wasn't a study book for the COMLEX, but the USMLE and COMLEX clinical skills exams were basically the same, except the COMLEX also tested OMT skills. The book had 100 high-yield minicases organized by chief complaint and 31 full-length cases that simulated the exam experience. When Dr. Patel had lulls between patients, I sat in her office and studied.

On Thursday of my second week, I drove six hours to Nashville, Tennessee, to stay overnight with a friend and his wife and four-month-old son. I had an interview at Vanderbilt on Friday! Vanderbilt's M.D. school had the cream of the crop, and I was a humble D.O. student. I was excited about the possibility of doing my psychiatry residency at Vanderbilt, but I wondered if I might feel dumb with all the big brains around me. My electronic residency application didn't show my COMLEX Level 2-PE result, and I decided not to talk about it unless asked. I planned to update my application after I received my retake result and transmit the results to the programs. Plenty of residency candidates wouldn't yet have their USMLE Step 2 CS or COMLEX Level 2-PE results if they took the exams later.

The Vanderbilt interview day was like the UofL day, but it also included a case presentation given by a resident for discussion. None of the faculty asked about my COMLEX Level 2-PE. All of the residents were Americans, and they appeared well-rested and happy. The facilities were also nice, of course. I drove home after lunch, arrived around 8 p.m., and happily told Lynn about my day.

I went on my Western interview tour December 1–9. Flights took me from Lexington, Kentucky, to Albuquerque, New Mexico; Salt Lake City, Utah; and Tucson, Arizona. I packed only a carry-on bag so I could travel efficiently and avoid checked bag fees and the risk of a checked bag getting lost. I wore my Columbia hooded ski jacket and packed my First Aid for the USMLE Step 2 CS book, one pair of jeans, two flannel shirts, dress shoes, a white Oxford shirt, tie, and my gray pinstripe wool suit. I booked hotels that had shuttle service so I wouldn't have to rent cars, and I only had to pay for my hotel in Utah. While I was on planes and waiting for planes, I diligently studied my book. And when I was in hotel rooms, I practiced writing patient notes under timed conditions. I enjoyed my whirlwind trip, and I kept in daily phone contact with Lynn to tell her about it. I met other residency candidates who were going on 12–20 interviews! I had only scheduled eight interviews because I figured that was enough to match with a program.

Most of the psychiatry residents at the University of New Mexico were happy Americans, and the facilities were nice. The program also had a unique moonlighting opportunity. Residents could take extra VA call shifts for $500, which sounded great to a poor medical student! A faculty member took the candidates for a 10-minute van ride to show us the Rio Grande Nature

Center State Park. The park was in a cottonwood bosque next to the Rio Grande River, and it offered a picturesque view of the snowy Sandia Mountains to the east.

All of the psychiatry residents at the University of Utah were happy Americans. The facilities were very nice and offered great views of the jagged, snowy Wasatch Mountains to the east. Salt Lake City was clean and beautiful, and it hosted the 2002 Winter Olympics. I stayed at the historic Peery Hotel downtown, and I enjoyed beer and delicious food at the Salty Dog Brewery across the street. When I had free time, I checked out the Mormon Temple Square Visitors' Center. I was glad I had my ski jacket because the temperature was 10 degrees and the cold stung my face when I walked from my hotel to Temple Square, which was a mile away. Visitors weren't allowed inside the temple, but the building, which took 40 years to build, looked impressive from the street. It reminded me of the Disney castle. I was excited about the possibility of doing my psychiatry residency at the University of Utah. World-class ski resorts were less than an hour away! There was only one snag with my Utah interview day: the program director asked about my COMLEX Level 2-PE result. I told him I failed the exam, but I was studying hard to retake it, and I would have the result about a month before Match Day.

The Southern Arizona University psychiatry residency was a new community-based program in Dillon, 20 minutes southeast of Tucson. The psychiatric hospital was adequate, but there was a plan to build a new psychiatric hospital and crisis center in less than two years. The crisis center would relieve pressure from the ED, which was often clogged with many psychiatric patients waiting for hospital beds. The program was so new that it didn't yet have fourth-year residents. Most of the residents were FMGs, but they all spoke English well, and they seemed happy. One of the FMGs was an American with an M.D. degree from a Caribbean medical school, and another FMG was a Dillon native who attended undergraduate school at SAU and medical school in Mexico. Interestingly, one of the third-year residents had been an anesthesiologist for 10 years. I met some other residency candidates on my interview trail who were also unhappy in other specialties.

The day after my Tucson interview, I flew back to Lexington and drove two and a half hours back to Brighton. I arrived around 6:30 p.m., exhausted from a long day of travel. Lynn gave me a big hug and kiss when I entered our apartment.

"I missed you!" she said.

"I missed you too, babe," I said.

"I'm so proud of you."

"Thanks."

Lynn had prepared a wonderful dinner for my arrival: salmon, sweet onions, and garlic roasted with a soy sauce and brown sugar glaze, saffron rice, steamed broccoli, and baby carrots. The meal and glass of cabernet were especially delicious after my long day. After dinner we watched a good movie, had hot sex, and fell into a deep sleep.

The next day, December 10, I continued to study for the COMLEX Level 2-PE, and in the evening I started my second ED rotation with an overnight shift. I worked overnight ED shifts until December 14, then took two days off before my exam. On December 16 I flew from Hansen, Tennessee, to Philadelphia. I was very thankful that my Aunt Martha, my father's sister, allowed me to use her Delta frequent flyer miles for the ticket! I stayed in a Marriott that was a 12-minute walk from the exam facility. The night before the exam, I relaxed. I turned on the TV, kicked back on the bed, and enjoyed a burger and fries delivered by room service and a Fat Tire amber ale. At bedtime I took half a milligram of Xanax from a new prescription. I hadn't taken the medication since the end of my second year of medical school. I called Lynn, and she wished me good luck. I prayed for God to help me pass the exam. My prayer life had improved since I failed the first exam, and family was also praying for me. I slept well.

Just enough of the Xanax was still in my system the next day to keep me from panicking without causing cognitive impairment, a common side effect. I prayed again before I started the exam. The experience was still nerve-wracking, of course, but I felt much better about my performance at the end of the day. Cold air hit me when I left the exam facility, and I was glad to return to the warm hotel. I called Lynn when I got to my room and told her I felt like I passed the exam.

"I told you you'd do better," she said. "Is your flight still on for tomorrow? They're canceling a bunch of flights because of that big storm."

"My flight's still scheduled for 10:15 in the morning," I said. "The storm isn't expected to hit Philadelphia until around midnight."

"Do you plan to stay in a hotel when you get to Hansen? I don't want you to drive on bad roads."

"I know how to drive in the snow. I lived in the Colorado Rockies for three years, and I had a rear-wheel drive car then. My car is a front-wheel drive. I'll just take it slow."

"We're expected to get 12 to 20 inches of accumulation."

"I know."

"I miss you, and I want you home, but I really don't want you to drive on bad roads. You may know how to drive, but there will be other idiots on the road. Please stay in a hotel."

"I'll be fine, babe. I'll be really careful."

"Call me when you get to Hansen."

"Okay. I love you."

"I love you too."

I turned on the TV, kicked back on the bed, and enjoyed seafood fettuccine Alfredo delivered by room service and two Fat Tires. I watched the Weather Channel for a little while. I was amused by how excited the meteorologists were to be covering the great blizzard of 2009. These were the moments they lived for, especially Jim Cantore, who relished being on location in the middle of storms, including hurricanes. He was bundled up in a blue parka in Boone, North Carolina, in the Appalachian Mountains.

The real adventure began the next day. My flight was delayed due to a mechanical problem. The plane needed a part that would be delivered on another plane. Hours passed as the departure time changed again and again, but the flight wasn't canceled. Some passengers became angry, and the waiting area thinned. But I decided to wait, even though I would miss my connection in Atlanta, because all of the next day's departures from Philadelphia were canceled. I called Lynn to update her. She told me it was snowing heavily in Brighton, and she pleaded with me again to stay another night in a hotel. The airplane part was finally installed, and the nearly empty plane departed at 10 p.m., just ahead of the storm.

I arrived in Atlanta after 12 a.m., and I spent a very uncomfortable night in the airport because I needed to talk to an agent at 6 a.m. about getting on a flight to Hansen. All of the chairs had armrests, so I couldn't lie down across chairs. I tried to recline in a chair with my feet on my carry-on bag, but it was very difficult to nap. I always had difficulty napping in airports and on planes. I got on a flight that departed for Hansen at 2:15 p.m.

When I finally arrived at the small regional airport in Hansen at 3:25 p.m., the sky was gray, and the landscape was covered with snow, but snow was no longer falling. I was bleary-eyed and running on fumes. I got a hot cup of coffee and called Lynn to let her know I arrived. She told me to be careful, and I headed to my car. The parking lot had been plowed, but I trudged through foot-deep snow around my car. I pulled my hands into my jacket sleeves and wiped snow off the windshield and windows with my forearms because I didn't have a brush or gloves. I got into the car, started the engine, turned the climate control to full heat, and cranked up the rock 'n' roll from my iPod. The temperature was 22 degrees, according to my car's thermometer. I hit the gas a little hard to back out of the parking spot because a pile of snow was behind my back bumper. Snow crunched underneath the car and tires.

The driving conditions woke me up before the coffee, which was too hot to sip at first. The route to Brighton was four lanes all the way through Tennessee, Virginia, and Kentucky, and it went through the Appalachian Mountains, so there were plenty of sections with significant inclines and curves with steep embankments. As soon as I left the airport, I noticed wrecked and stuck vehicles in deep snow off the sides of the road and in the median. As I continued to drive, I noticed more abandoned vehicles. I was one of the few moving vehicles on the road, which was fine with me. The drive demanded my full attention, even when I was only going 30–45 miles per hour. It was difficult to tell where the road was at times, especially as the gray sky grew dimmer. I kept my car in whichever lane had the least snow, and sometimes I drove in the middle of the road. Sometimes snow scraped the bottom of my car, the car slid, and my front tires spun. I passed abandoned pileups and wrecked semitrucks, and some of them were in my northbound lanes. I saw vehicles sliding and spinning around, going off the road. Some idiots were going too fast, and I watched some of them wreck, including drivers in big pickup trucks and SUVs who were probably overconfident. The only time I went a little faster was when I approached inclines to keep my momentum up to get to the top, then I slowed down as I drove down the other side. I stopped counting abandoned vehicles after I reached 100 about halfway through my trip. After an hour and a half of driving, only my headlights illuminated the hazardous road.

The trip from Hansen to Brighton normally took two hours, but the white-knuckle driving took three and a half hours. I finally arrived in Brighton around 7 p.m., but, unfortunately, the adventure wasn't over. The storm had knocked out electricity to parts of the town, and Lynn was bundled up in our cold, dark apartment. She greeted me with a flashlight, and I could see her breath.

"I'm so glad you're home!" She gave me a big hug and kiss. "Our power's been out since last night."

"That sucks," I said. "I'm sorry."

"Yeah. I'm freezing, and we don't have hot water either. I haven't had a shower in two days."

"If power's on at the medical school, we could use the anatomy lab showers in the basement. Have you eaten?"

"No. I'm starving too! I'm so glad you came home tonight."

"Me too. Why don't we get something to eat in a warm restaurant, and I'll see if the showers have hot water?"

"That sounds great!"

We left the apartment with some toiletries, towels, and clean clothes. Lights were on at the Waffle House, so we had bacon, eggs, and hash browns for dinner, which was especially satisfying! Lights were also on at BCSOM. I still had a key to the medical school, even though I hadn't needed it since my first-year anatomy course. I unlocked the only door to the basement, which was in the middle of the hall, and headed to the men's showers. The hall was lined with lockers, and it was dark, only illuminated by exit signs at the door and left end of the hall, which had stairs leading to the foyer at the top of the first-year lecture hall. It was kind of creepy being alone in the dark basement at night with the cadavers. The showers had hot water, and we felt much better after we took hot showers.

The power was still out when we returned to our icy apartment. We lit some candles in our living room, and I fired up my camping lantern and stove as Lynn worried about me burning down the apartment or poisoning us with carbon monoxide. We sat next to each other on the couch, bundled up, and we warmed our hands by the lantern and stove on the coffee table in front of us. Thankfully, one of Lynn's friends called to let her know that a second-year medical student was out of town for Christmas break, and he didn't mind us staying in his downtown apartment, which had power. We called the student, and he told us we could get a key from his landlord. We expressed our heartfelt gratitude, grabbed some belongings and a bottle of cabernet, which wasn't frozen, and we enjoyed a cold glass of cabernet in the warm second-story apartment before going to sleep.

I resumed my ED rotation in the morning. Lynn called to let me know power was back on at our apartment, and she was going to bake cookies for the student. I worked ED shifts until an overnight Christmas Eve/Christmas Day shift, and I had the rest of Christmas Day and the day after off. I slept part of Christmas day away, then we opened presents, talked with family on the phone, and enjoyed a delicious dinner of honey ham, green beans, garlic mashed potatoes, and sautéed cinnamon apples. I returned to the ED on December 27 and continued to work until New Year's Eve. I returned home shortly after 7 p.m., exhausted, and Lynn and I had pizza for dinner. She always liked to watch the ball drop in New York City at midnight, but I couldn't stay awake after two glasses of Asti. She didn't have to work the next day, but I did.

Endnotes

1. Match Day occurs on the third Friday of March each year when the National Resident Matching Program (NRMP) releases residency placement results to fourth-year medical students and FMGs. An algorithm determines where applicants match, based on how programs and applicants rank each other, and both parties are contractually bound to accept the results. About 94% of U.S. medical graduates match on the first try, and an additional 3% find a residency during the "scramble" that starts on Black Monday before Match Day. Only about 50% of FMGs match with programs.

Chapter 19

Neurology

I started my elective neurology rotation with Apoorva Trivedi, M.D., on Friday, New Year's Day, with a distracting champagne headache. Her clinic was located in a narrow, gray brick building in a run-down area on the south side of downtown Brighton. She shared the clinic with her husband, Munish, who was a pain management physician. Dr. Trivedi was an FMG with a medical degree from India, and she had completed a four-year neurology residency in the U.S.

I arrived at the clinic at 8 a.m. A shady-looking man and woman were sitting in the small waiting area just inside the entrance. At least there wasn't a line of shady-looking people stretching out into the street as there was at Dr. Hoover's pill mill in Williamson, West Virginia. The inside of the clinic needed a fresh, lighter coat of paint and brighter lights. The sides of the building had no windows; only the front entrance had a large glass window and glass door. Dr. Trivedi met me at the front desk. She appeared middle-aged, attractive, and well-dressed.

"Dr. Trivedi. Good morning," I said. "I'm James Banks."

"Welcome, James," she said with an exotic accent. "How are you this morning?"

"Good. How are you?"

"Good, thank you. I heard you're going into psychiatry."

"Yes. I've interviewed for six residencies, and I have two more interviews this month."

"That's exciting. Do you have your top choice yet?"

"Not yet. I'll figure that out after I finish my interviews."

"Well, I hope your last interviews go well."

"Thank you."

I saw seven patients with paresthesia, neuropathy, extremity weakness, trigeminal neuralgia, and tremor. The patient with paresthesia was a 34-year-old female who had tingling sensations in her left upper and lower extremities and right lower abdomen, and she appeared worried. The tingling started with her left leg a few months earlier, and symptoms improved. But a month later she had tingling in her left arm and abdomen, and the symptoms worsened. She denied numbness, weakness, muscle cramps, tremor, dizziness, difficulty with walking or talking, changes in vision, cognitive problems, bladder or bowel problems, but she complained of fatigue.

I conducted a head-to-toe neurological exam. For the cranial nerve exam, I had her follow my finger with her eyes to check extraocular movement; I checked her pupil responses with a penlight, and I had her squeeze her eyelids tightly shut, raise her eyebrows, blow out her cheeks, smile, clench her teeth as I palpated her jaw muscles, stick out her tongue and say "ahhh," shrug her shoulders, and turn her head from side to side against my resistance. I checked light touch sensation in her face, upper and lower extremities, and I checked strength and reflexes in her upper and lower extremities. I checked vibration sensation by placing a vibrating tuning fork on the joints of her great toes. I had her stand and close her eyes to check for a Romberg sign (loss of balance). I observed her gait. Her exam was normal, except for decreased light touch sensation in her left leg and decreased vibration sensation in her left toe.

Dr. Trivedi agreed with my exam findings, and she also evaluated coordination by having the patient perform rapidly alternating and point-to-point movements. The patient placed her hands on her thighs, then rapidly turned her hands over and raised them, and she repeated the movement about a dozen times without difficulty. She touched her nose with her right index finger, then touched Dr. Trivedi's outstretched finger with the same finger a few times. She did this a few more times with her eyes closed. She repeated the movement with her other hand, and she had no difficulty with either hand. She lay supine on the exam table, placed her right heel on her left shin just below the knee, and slid it down the shin to the top of the foot. She quickly repeated the movement a few times with both feet, and she didn't have a problem with either foot. Dr. Trivedi also tested position sense by having the patient close her eyes and report if her large toe was up or down when Dr. Trivedi moved the toe. Her position sense was intact.

Dr. Trivedi scheduled her for a somatosensory evoked potentials study. If the test were to show delayed sensory nerve conduction, a brain MRI would be ordered to look for demyelinating lesions—signs of MS, an autoimmune inflammatory disease that attacks myelinated axons (nerve fibers) in the brain and spinal cord. Myelin is a fatty substance that forms thick sheaths around the axons of some neurons (nerve cells) and insulates the axons to speed electrical impulses.

I was happy that Dr. Trivedi was done seeing patients by noon. My headache hadn't improved with ibuprofen. I returned home, took a small dose of Benadryl, drank some water, and took a nap. I was relieved to awaken without a headache. I was very tired after working five 12-hour ED shifts and half a day in the neurology clinic, so I vegetated over the weekend. On Saturday morning when Lynn and I returned to our apartment with groceries, we saw Elsie's nephew and another young man moving boxes and furniture out of her upstairs apartment.

"We didn't know Elsie was moving," Lynn said.

"She passed away," her nephew said.

"Oh, I'm so sorry to hear that," Lynn said. "When did she die?"

"A couple of weeks ago."

"We knew she had heart problems."

"Yeah," I said. "I saw her in the cardiology clinic a few months ago, and she said she had been to the ER because her defibrillator shocked her a few times in the middle of the night."

"Well, I guess her heart finally gave out," he said.

"She was really frail, but I can't believe she's gone," Lynn said. "She was a good neighbor."

"She was a good aunt too. I could never understand why her daughter wouldn't have anything to do with her. She didn't even attend the funeral. I guess getting high was more important to her."

"That's really sad," Lynn said.

"Yes, it is," I said. "Could you guys use a hand?"

"We've got it, thanks. She didn't have much stuff."

"Okay. Well, we're sorry for your loss," I said.

"Yes," Lynn said. "We'll really miss her. She was so sweet."

"Thank you. I'll miss her too."

Lynn became tearful when we entered the apartment. "That's so sad."

"Yeah. It sounds like her daughter's a piece of shit."

"What kind of daughter wouldn't go to her own mother's funeral?"

"The kind who's addicted to drugs. It is very sad."

Dr. Trivedi was off on Monday, so I read about MS.

On Tuesday I saw a 49-year-old female with diabetic polyneuropathy and chronic ataxia (incoordination) due to idiopathic cerebellar degeneration, a rare disease. She had significant difficulty walking, talking, feeding, and dressing herself. I also saw my first-year biochemistry professor, Dr. Faulkner. He was 55 years old, and he had parkinsonism, a disease caused by degeneration of dopaminergic neurons deep in the brain. He was sitting in a chair in an exam room with his head downcast, and he had a cane next to him. He appeared slim, handsome, clean-shaven, with a full head of brown hair, well-dressed.

"Good morning, Dr. Faulkner," I said.

"Good morning, James," He could only raise his head a little bit, and he had difficulty making eye contact. His affect was flat. "How are your rotations going?"

"Good, thanks." I sat down on a stool, and it was easier for him to make eye contact. "It's been a while. I'm sorry to see you again under these circumstances."

"Me too."

"Does your neck hurt? That looks really uncomfortable."

"It is uncomfortable. Sometimes it really bothers me, and I get headaches. Botox injections help, but the last treatment hasn't lasted as long."

"When did you get your last injections?"

"Two months ago."

"And you're taking Sinemet?"[1]

"Yes."

"How's the medication working for you?"

"It helps. I tried a higher dose, but I couldn't tolerate it. I had nausea, and I went a little crazy."

"What do you mean by a little crazy?"

"I was confused, and I started having hallucinations."

"What kind of hallucinations?"

"I saw some angels. I had to cancel class one day. I called Dr. Trivedi, and she advised me to decrease the dose."

"Are you still teaching?"

"Yes. I plan to keep doing that as long as I can."

"Are you still doing photography when you have time?"

"Yes. I got a right-angle viewfinder so I can look down at the camera."

"Well, I'm glad you're still able to teach and photograph. Have you had any falls?"

"No. I had a near fall, but I was able to catch myself."

"I see you have a pill-rolling tremor in your right hand."

"Yeah. It comes and goes."

"Stretch your arms out in front of you."

The tremor resolved with his outstretched arms.

"Okay," I said. "Now touch your nose with your right index finger, then touch my finger."

The movement didn't cause an action tremor. I flexed and extended his forearms while palpating his biceps and triceps. The muscles were rigid, resistant to passive movement.

"Let me see how you walk in the hall," I said.

He had difficulty rising from his seat. He was able to stand after the third attempt. "It takes me a moment to get going." His posture was stooped, and he stood still for a moment. He took a few stuttering steps toward the door. I grabbed his cane and handed it to him. His stuttering resolved in the hall, but his gait was slow and shuffling. We returned to the room, and he sat in the chair.

"I'm glad to see you're using a cane, but it looks like you need to start using a walker," I said.

"Dr. Trivedi and my family doc told me the same thing, but I'm not ready for that," he said. "Old people in nursing homes use walkers. I'm really careful."

"Okay. But what if you start to fall to the left, and your cane's in your right hand?"

"Then I guess I'm screwed." He laughed.

I smiled. "I'm glad to see you have a sense of humor. I'm really sorry you're having to deal with this. I'll pray for you."

"Thank you. I can't imagine how hard it would be to cope with this without my faith."

Dr. Faulkner declined Dr. Trivedi's offer to increase Sinemet, and Dr. Trivedi told him she would see if she could get insurance approval to give him Botox injections one month early.

After I was done in the clinic, I saw six patients in the hospital. Four of them had strokes. A 63-year-old female couldn't move her left upper extremity. She could move her left lower extremity but not fully against gravity.

On Wednesday in the clinic, I saw patients with migraines, seizure disorders, cervical dystonia, fibromyalgia, and radiculopathy (pain, numbness, weakness) due to disc herniations. A 49-year-old female had migraines since she had been kicked in the head by a horse one and a half years earlier.

Some migraines were debilitating, caused nausea and vomiting, and she had to lie in her dark bedroom all day. I advised her to consider trying the OMT clinic at BCSOM or BMC to see if manipulation could help to relieve her symptoms. After I was done in the clinic, I saw two hospital cases.

On Thursday I drove four hours to Winston-Salem, North Carolina, to stay overnight with Lynn's parents. I had an interview at Wake Forest on Friday! Wake Forest was a prestigious institution like Vanderbilt. All of the residents were happy Americans, and the facilities were nice. The program director asked about my COMLEX Level 2-PE result. I told her I had to retake the exam, and I would have the result about a month before Match Day. I drove home after lunch, arrived around 5:30 p.m., and happily told Lynn about my day.

On Tuesday morning I drove two and a half hours to Lexington for a 1 p.m. interview with the University of Kentucky. I had to tell the program director about my COMLEX Level 2-PE issue. The facilities were tired, and I didn't get good vibes from the residents. They were nice, but they didn't appear happy, and half of them were FMGs. I enjoyed a sushi dinner with some of the residents, compliments of the psychiatry department, and I learned that two of them had scrambled into the program— another bad sign. I drove home after dinner, arrived around 8:30 p.m., and told Lynn that UK would probably be at the bottom of my residency rank order list.

On Wednesday in the clinic I saw a 36-year-old female with post-concussion syndrome (left-sided headache, dizziness, concentration difficulty) and depression. She had sustained a left skull fracture and epidural hematoma from a motor vehicle accident one and a half years earlier. She was an unrestrained passenger in a car that was struck by a train. I advised her to consider trying the OMT clinic at BCSOM or BMC.

After I was done in the clinic, I saw an interesting hospital case. Ms. Cantrell was 70 years old, and she was catatonic. She had been admitted for pneumonia and respiratory failure. After she was extubated she talked during the first 24 hours, then she stopped talking, and she didn't appear to be concerned. Her room was dim, and she was sitting up in bed, staring blankly ahead. She appeared older than her stated age.

"Ms. Cantrell. Good afternoon," I said. "I'm James. I'm a medical student working with Dr. Trivedi, a neurologist who has been consulted to see you."

She looked at me but didn't speak.

"How are you feeling?" I said.

She didn't respond.

"I understand you were admitted for pneumonia and breathing failure, and you were talking for a while after your breathing tube was pulled out, but you stopped talking yesterday."

She didn't nod or shake her head.

"Could you tell me how you're doing in writing?" I handed her my pocket notebook and a pen.

She held the notebook and pen but didn't write anything.

"Okay. Well, I need to examine you."

She followed my directions to examine her cranial nerves and strength in her upper and lower extremities, and I checked her reflexes. Strength and reflexes were normal, and she walked without difficulty. Dr. Trivedi examined her and asked if she had any recent stress or past trauma in her life, but she didn't respond. Dr. Trivedi privately told me she probably had conversion disorder, a mental disorder in which psychological conflict causes alteration in voluntary motor or sensory functioning.

On Thursday Ms. Cantrell still wasn't talking or writing, but she was otherwise cooperative and followed directions. I saw several interesting patients in the clinic.

A 51-year-old female complained of low back pain and a left leg injury from a fall. She had been on workers' compensation since age 42, disability since age 43, and her disability case had recently come under review. She also saw psychiatrist Dr. Damron. She had worked as an RN at Luray Behavioral Health Center until an agitated patient assaulted her and injured her back. She developed PTSD, and workers' comp covered her neurological and psychiatric care. X-rays of her back and leg didn't show any obvious injuries. Aside from the back pain, numbness, tingling, and weakness in her left leg, she had a range of other complaints. Her neurological exam was normal, except she reported decreased light-touch sensation. Dr. Trivedi suspected she was malingering because she was worried about losing her disability.

A 31-year-old female had balance difficulty and blurry vision. A brain MRI showed a lesion on her cerebellum, and her cerebrospinal fluid (CSF) was normal, so she was scheduled for an evoked potential study to rule out MS.

Mr. Eldridge was a 63-year-old civil engineer who had major personality changes and declining cognition over the past three months. Mr. Eldridge and his wife were sitting in chairs in an exam room. Mr. Eldridge appeared his stated age, balding, overweight, clean-shaven, well-dressed. His wife appeared stressed.

"Mr. Eldridge. Good morning," I said. "I'm James. I'm a medical student working with Dr. Trivedi."

"Good morning," he said. "Who's Dr. Trivedi?"

"She's a neurologist."

"Why am I seeing a neurologist?"

"Your wife has been concerned about you having personality changes and problems with your memory over the last few months."

"I don't know why she'd say that. There's nothing wrong with me. I really don't need to be here, but she insisted I see a doctor. If my wife's not happy, nobody's happy, if you know what I mean."

"I do know what you mean. It's the same way with my wife." I smiled, and he smiled back. "You're a civil engineer?"

"Yes."

"How have you been doing at work?"

"Work was going fine, but I decided to take some time off."

"Why did you decide to take time off?"

"I just needed a vacation."

"How long have you been off work?"

"For a while."

"How long is a while?"

"I can't say exactly. I don't really keep track of time."

"Do you know what day of the week it is?"

"No. I really haven't been keeping track of the days since I've been off work."

"Do you know the date?"

"No."

"How about the month?"

"January."

"Year?"

"Two thousand ten."

"Season?"

"Winter."

"What city and state are you in?"

"Branham, Kentucky."

"You're actually in Brighton."

"Okay. My wife drove me here. I wasn't paying attention to where she was going."

"Do you know the name of this place where you are?"

"I know I'm at a doctor's office, but I don't know the name of the clinic."

"What floor are you on?"

"Is that a trick question? Isn't this a one-story building?"

"I guess it is a trick question. This is a one-story building. Why do you think your wife would be concerned about you having personality changes?"

"I have no idea. I'm my same old self."

His wife said, "He's been gambling, going to bars, and he drove all the way to Lexington to go to a strip club."

"What's wrong with having a little fun?" he said. "She's just a fuddy-duddy."

"He never had any of this behavior before. We've been married for 40 years, and he never had a drop of alcohol until recently. He's an elder at our church."

"What's wrong with having some drinks and getting some action on the side when your wife doesn't put out anymore? A man's got needs."

"He has never talked like this either."

"She doesn't care about my needs because she's been getting it on with another man."

"There isn't another man."

"I have proof."

"What proof? You've never been able to show me any proof."

"Well, I have it."

"He didn't decide to take a vacation either. His boss told him to take off work and see a doctor because he was acting strange and he couldn't complete his tasks."

"There were no problems with my work. I just needed to take some time off."

"He's also talked to people who aren't really there. He's wet his pants. He gets up in the middle of the night, wanders around the house, and rummages through things. One night he was digging through the garbage. Another night he was in the attic. He gets upset and angry easily."

"Of course I got angry when I found out you started banging another man."

"I've always been faithful to you, honey."

"Are there any firearms in the house?" I said.

"His son took them," his wife said.

"Good," I said.

Dr. Trivedi ordered a brain MRI to look for atrophy of frontal and temporal lobes, signs of frontotemporal dementia.

On Friday Ms. Cantrell still wasn't talking, but she was no longer in the hospital when I returned on Monday. In the clinic I saw Ms. Stanley, a 45-year-old disabled female with fibromyalgia who complained of right foot numbness and left-sided numbness and weakness. She appeared older than her stated age, disheveled, and she had a range of other physical complaints, including generalized pain, fatigue, headaches, dizziness, nausea, diarrhea, and constipation. She was very concerned about all of her symptoms, and she was frustrated by other doctors being unable to find anything physically wrong with her. She wasn't satisfied with her family medicine doctor because he didn't order enough labs and tests, so she found an internist who ordered a range of labs and tests. She had monthly visits with the internist, and he referred her to other specialists, including a rheumatologist, gastroenterologist, ENT (ear nose throat) doctor, neurologist, and psychiatrist.

Dr. Trivedi examined her and asked if she had any recent stress or past trauma in her life. She denied stress but admitted that she had been sexually abused when she was a child. She had been raised by her alcoholic mother, who had different boyfriends when she was growing up. Dr. Trivedi asked how her mother responded to her when she was upset as a child. Her mother told her to "shut up. Quit crying."

"I'm sorry you had such a difficult and traumatic childhood," Dr. Trivedi said. "Your neurological exam is normal. Some of your symptoms could be caused by emotional distress, especially since your mother didn't help you verbalize your emotions when you were a child. When you cried she should have asked you why you were upset to help you put your emotions into words, instead of telling you to shut up and stop crying. When you don't have words associated with emotions, the emotions can manifest as physical symptoms."

"You're saying this is all in my head!" she said.

"I'm not saying your symptoms aren't real. I'm sure your symptoms are very real, and they're causing significant problems for you, but I don't have a neurological diagnosis for you."

"Well, can't you order some tests, like scan my head, test my nerves?"

"I have reviewed records from your internist and other specialists. You have had many labs and tests, and your brain MRI was normal four months ago."

"Can't you do other tests? Maybe I need another MRI. Maybe something was missed with the other MRI."

"I'm sorry. I can't justify ordering more tests, based on your exam."

"So you can't help me either?"

"I recommend you keep your appointment with the psychiatrist."

"I'm not crazy."

"I'm not saying you're crazy, but a psychiatrist may be able to help you with your emotions, and he could refer you to a psychotherapist. Talk therapy could help you develop emotional awareness and work through past trauma."

"Maybe the psychiatrist can order another MRI."

After the appointment Dr. Trivedi told me she appeared to have somatization disorder.

I saw more patients with MS, a 19-year-old female with left leg weakness and disease onset at age 13, a 37-year-old female with chronic gait ataxia, and a 33-year-old female with chronic ataxia that affected her upper and lower extremities. I also saw Mr. Hunt, a 52-year-old male with Huntington disease, a rare, inherited autosomal dominant disease characterized by neurodegeneration deep in the brain, chorea (irregular, spasmodic involuntary movement of the limbs and facial muscles), dementia, and psychiatric disorders. Symptoms usually begin in the 30s or 40s, and the disease is relentlessly progressive, resulting in death after an average course of about 15 years.

Mr. Hunt was in a wheelchair in an exam room with his morbidly obese wife in a chair beside him. Mr. Hunt appeared older than his stated age, well-groomed, with gray hair, casually dressed. He had jerking, writhing movements of his head, upper and lower extremities. It was painful to observe. I felt strong empathy for him.

"Mr. Hunt. Hello," I said. "I'm James. I'm a medical student working with Dr. Trivedi."

"Hi," he said.

"How are you?"

"Okay."

"That sounds like a polite answer. How are you really doing?"

"I'm managing as best I can, and I've been blessed with a wonderful wife." He suddenly became emotional and cried loudly.

"I've been blessed with a wonderful husband," his wife said. She put a hand on his leg.

"I don't know why God is punishing me!" He sobbed.

"God's not punishing you, darling. You're a good man."

"I must be a terrible man to have this fucking disease!" he said angrily. "I wish God would just go ahead and take me and end my suffering!"

"I'm sorry, honey. He never used to curse before this terrible disease took hold of him. We're Christians."

"Do you attend a church?" I said.

"Oh, yes," she said. "We still go regularly, even though he has to use a wheelchair, unless he's having a really bad day. I don't know what we'd do without our church. They've been praying for us."

"I know suicide is wrong, but I've thought about it," he said, crying. "I'm useless now, and my wife has to take care of me. I hate being on disability."

"He was a contractor for 27 years. He built big, beautiful homes for doctors. And he never had emotional problems before. He was never depressed, and he never talked about suicide."

"I'm sorry both of you are having to deal with this," I said. "This is a devastating disease."

He laughed loudly.

"His moods change on a dime now as you can see," she said.

"Are you taking your Celexa and Lamictal?" I said.

"Yes," he said.

"Maybe Dr. Trivedi could adjust medication to help with mood stability," I said.

"That would be great," she said.

"I'm glad you have the support of your church. I'll pray for you too."

They both said, "Thank you."

Dr. Trivedi increased Lamictal.

During my last week I saw a couple of interesting patients in the clinic. A 22-year-old coal miner sustained an electric shock injury five months earlier, and he had low back pain, leg pain, weakness, myoclonic jerks (involuntary muscle contractions), and balance difficulty. A 45-year-old female had vertigo, bilateral lower extremity and left upper extremity weakness, paresthesia, and burning pain for two weeks; and right upper extremity weakness and paresthesia for two days, following an influenza vaccination three weeks earlier. She had difficulty walking and reflexes were diminished, so Dr. Trivedi admitted her to BMC for Guillain-Barré syndrome, a rare demyelinating polyneuropathy of rapid onset that usually develops after a respiratory or gastrointestinal viral illness but can rarely occur after vaccination. The syndrome classically causes ascending paralysis that begins with the lower extremities and can involve the upper extremities, respiratory muscles, and cranial nerves. The patient's CSF showed increased protein as expected, and a brain MRI showed periventricular white matter gliosis, which was unexpected and could be a sign of MS. She received IV immunoglobulin (IVIG), and she was still in the hospital on my last day.

I also saw a repeat visitor in the hospital. Ms. Blair was 39 years old, and she had MS and schizoaffective disorder. She was sitting up in bed, watching TV. She appeared older than her stated age, disheveled, with blonde hair, casually dressed. When I saw her during my hospitalist rotation 11 months earlier, she had an MS pseudoexacerbation after she broke up with her alcoholic boyfriend of two to three months.

"Ms. Blair. Good afternoon," I said. "I'm James."

"I remember you," she said.

"Yes. I saw you in February of last year when I was on a hospitalist rotation. I'm working with Dr. Trivedi now."

"Dr. Trivedi is great. So you've decided to become a neurologist?"

"No. I'm just doing a neurology rotation. Medical students have to rotate through different specialties."

"What kind of doctor are you going to be then?"

"Psychiatrist."

"Cool. I've got a psychiatrist too, and he's a good one, thank God, 'cause I've had some real quacks over the years."

"I'm sorry to hear that."

"It's okay. I've managed. I think you'll be a good psychiatrist."

"Thank you. So what brought you to the hospital this time?"

"I started having problems with my legs again."

"What kind of problems?"

"They just felt like they were giving out on me."

"Did you fall?"

"I almost did, but, thankfully, I was close to the couch, so I just sat down."

"Well, I'm glad you didn't fall."

"Me too."

"When did your legs start to give out?"

"Yesterday."

"How were you doing before this happened?"

"I was really sad because I had to put my Snookums to sleep."

"I'm sorry to hear that. Was Snookums your dog?"

"Yes, and he was my best friend." She became tearful. "I'm a wreck without him. He was my emotional support animal."

"Do you have anyone else for support?"

"No. I don't talk to my family, and I decided to stay away from men for a while. I don't know why I always seem to end up with the bad ones."

"Why don't you talk to your family?"

"My mom and sister are crazier than me. They're always stirring up trouble, so it's best for me to just stay away from them. I don't need any more drama in my life."

"Okay. Could you swing your legs over the side of the bed?" I examined strength, sensation, and reflexes in her lower and upper extremities. "Let's see how you walk in the hall."

She walked without difficulty. "I still feel a little weak, but I think I'm doing better."

"Good."

Dr. Trivedi examined her, advised her to follow up with her in the clinic, and she was discharged.

On Friday I thanked Dr. Trivedi for the experience, and she gave me a good evaluation.

Endnotes

1. Sinemet is a combination of levodopa and carbidopa. Levodopa is converted to dopamine in the brain, and carbidopa prevents dopamine from being metabolized before it reaches the brain.

Chapter 20

Neurosurgery

I started my elective neurosurgery rotation with Raymond Jackson, M.D., and Peter Wilson, M.D., in February. Both doctors had completed grueling seven-year residencies to become brain and spine surgeons, and BMC was proud to employ them. Not surprisingly, neither doctor was married. Such a career path left very little room for life outside of work.

On Monday at 7:15 a.m., I changed into scrubs in the OR men's locker room, and I met Dr. Jackson in the OR doctors' lounge. He was standing, sipping a cup of coffee, socializing with Dr. Davis, the general surgeon I rotated with. Dr. Jackson was young, black, handsome, clean-shaven, muscular, wearing green scrubs.

"What are you doing here?" Dr. Davis said to me.

"Nice to see you too," I said. "I'm here to meet Dr. Jackson."

"Well, he's pretty easy to spot," Dr. Davis said.

"Mark thinks he's a funny guy," Dr. Jackson said. "Man, you're tall."

"That's what I've been told." I said. "I'm James Banks."

"Good morning, James," Dr. Jackson said. He smiled brightly and gave me a strong handshake.

"So you've changed your mind and decided to become a brain surgeon?" Dr. Davis said.

"No. I thought neurosurgery would be an interesting elective," I said.

"What are you going into?" Dr. Jackson said.

"Psychiatry."

"No shit!"

"Yeah."

"I had a crazy grandma. She was bipolar or schizophrenic or something. I guess that means I've got a little crazy in me."

"You've probably got a loose screw or two," Dr. Davis said.

"Doesn't everybody have a loose screw or two?" Dr. Jackson said.

"I don't know. Do they?" I said.

"You're a funny guy too," Dr. Jackson said. "Come on, you've got to be a little crazy to go into psychiatry, right?"

"Maybe."

"Well, I don't have the patience to deal with crazy people. When I did my inpatient psych rotation in medical school, I told a patient he was terrible at suicide because he had tried to kill himself three times, but he was still alive."

We laughed.

"The attending psychiatrist didn't appreciate my comment," Dr. Jackson said. "Okay. So you wanna see some neurosurgery?"

"Yeah," I said.

"Well, I hope this will be a good rotation for you. Your first day will be easy. We just have a lumbar discectomy this morning."

"Okay."

We scrubbed, and I observed Dr. Jackson operate on an obese 29-year-old female who was prone (face down) on the operating table. I didn't mind that I wasn't allowed to assist with the surgery. Dr. Jackson wore a headset with glasses, a light, and binocular loupes for the delicate surgery. A small incision was made to the right of the lumbar spine, and electrocautery was used to stop bleeding. Fascia and muscles were resected and retracted to reveal the L4 and L5 vertebral laminae and ligamentum flavum that form the posterior of the spinal canal. Laminae are flat plates of bone, and the ligamentum flavum is a ligament that binds together the laminae of adjoining vertebrae. A bent needle was placed in the L4–5 disc to confirm the level with an x-ray. Part of the L4 lamina was removed with a burr (small rotary cutting tool) and Kerrison punch. The ligamentum flavum was gently resected, and the dural sac and nerves were gently retracted. The dural sac is a continuation of the spinal dura mater below the termination of the spinal cord (L1–2 level). The spinal dura mater is a strong, membranous sheath that surrounds the spinal cord and cauda equina and is continuous with the cranial dura mater. The cauda equina is a bundle of nerves at the end of the spinal cord that resembles a horse's tail. The disc herniation was removed, and the wound was closed.

We didn't have any surgical cases on Tuesday. I arrived at BMC's shiny neurosurgery clinic at 8 a.m. The building was located across the street from BMC. A Porsche 911 and Audi R8 supercar were in the parking lot. The front desk receptionist led me to a large, shared doctors' office in the back of the clinic. Dr. Jackson and Dr. Wilson were sitting at desks with computers on opposite sides of the room, facing each other. Dr. Wilson appeared young, slim, clean-shaven, wearing a white lab coat, white Oxford shirt, and khaki pants.

"Good morning," I said.

"Good morning," Dr. Jackson said. "James, this is my partner, Dr. Wilson."

"Dr. Wilson, nice to meet you," I said.

"Likewise." Dr. Wilson stood and shook my hand.

"He's gonna be a psychiatrist," Dr. Jackson said.

"No shit," Dr. Wilson said.

"That's what I said," Dr. Jackson said.

"What made you decide to do a neurosurgery rotation?" Dr. Wilson said.

"I thought it would be interesting," I said. "My neuroscience and neurology courses were really interesting, and I did a neurology rotation last month."

"Okay. Well, we've never had a future psychiatrist rotate with us before. Welcome."

"Thank you."

"We have another easy day today," Dr. Jackson said. "It's a slow clinic day."

The first patient was Mr. Nichols, a 47-year-old male with neck pain. Dr. Jackson and I went to the back corner of a hall to review the cervical MRI on a large computer screen. He used the mouse to scroll through sagittal and transverse images.

"What do you see here?" Dr. Jackson said.

"Is that a disc herniation at C6–C7?" I said.

"Yes. It's a small one. What else?"

"Are these disc bulges above the herniation?"

"Yes."

We entered the exam room. Mr. Nichols was sitting in a chair. He appeared older than his stated age.

"Good morning, Mr. Nichols," Dr. Jackson said. "I have a student with me today. This is James." Dr. Jackson sat on a rolling stool.

"Nice to meet you," I said.

"Nice to meet you," Mr. Nichols said.

"How are you, man?" Dr. Jackson said.

"I'm okay, except for my neck. The pain really gets to me sometimes, and my neck gets crackly, and I get bad headaches."

"Have you had pain, numbness, tingling, or weakness in your arms or hands?"

"No."

"Good. Let me check your strength. Grab my fingers and make tight fists."

Mr. Nichols made fists around Dr. Jackson's index and middle fingers.

"Good," Dr. Jackson said. He grabbed Mr. Nichols' wrists. "Push against me."

Mr. Nichols tried to extend his forearms against resistance. "You're strong."

Dr. Jackson smiled. "Okay. Now pull."

Mr. Nichols tried to flex his forearms against resistance. "I wouldn't want to arm wrestle you."

Dr. Jackson laughed and released his wrists. "Your MRI does show a small disc herniation at C6–C7, but it's not impinging on a nerve, and I don't recommend surgery. You're a smoker?"

"I'm trying to quit."

"Well, I hope you're able to quit 'cause smoking is terrible for your spine. It accelerates the development of degenerative disc disease and osteoporosis. Do you know what osteoporosis is?"

"My mom has that. She takes medicine to keep her bones strong."

"How old is your mom?"

"Seventy."

"Okay. Well, osteoporosis is bone loss. Eighty percent of people who get osteoporosis are postmenopausal women. It's a condition that affects old ladies and causes hip fractures. You're a 47-year-old man, so you should have pretty strong bones, but smoking increases your risk of having a spinal fracture by 32 percent."

"I didn't know that smoking was bad for my spine."

"Most people don't. Do you want to be like an old lady?"

"No."

"Of course not. You really need to quit smoking then. Otherwise, I will be cutting on your neck before long."

"I really don't want to have my neck cut on anyway."

"Good. Maybe that will motivate you to quit smoking. You can take ibuprofen or Tylenol as needed for pain."

"Tylenol and ibuprofen don't help much."

"You can talk to your primary care doctor about that. He may want to refer you to a pain management specialist. And you can try physical therapy. Would you like a referral for physical therapy?"

"Sure. I'll try anything that might help."

"Okay. We'll refer you."

"Thank you."

"You're welcome."

We left the room and saw three more patients. Dr. Jackson advised a 67-year-old obese male with low back pain to lose weight to relieve extra strain and pressure on his back, and he ordered an MRI. He advised a 49-year-old obese female with low back pain and a L4–5 synovial cyst to lose weight. The cyst was small, and she didn't have lower extremity radiculopathy, so he didn't recommend surgery. He also didn't recommend surgery for a 32-year-old female with a small cyst deep in her brain in the right lateral ventricle (CSF-filled cavity). The cyst was discovered incidentally with a head CT when she visited the ED for a severe headache with nausea and vomiting. Dr. Jackson advised her that the cyst was only 8 mm in the largest dimension, it wasn't obstructing CSF flow, and it wasn't the cause of her migraine.

On Tuesday afternoon I received a call from Dr. Anderson, inviting me and Lynn to have dinner with him and Dr. Vaswani on Saturday, and we gladly accepted the invitation. He told me Dr. Vaswani still had reservations about me potentially being a resident in the UNT psychiatry program, especially after some residents complained about me emailing them more questions after my interview. They said they answered all my questions on my interview day, and I asked too many questions.

On Wednesday I observed two surgeries. The first case was an open cranial biopsy for a 79-year-old female with a 2.2-cm mass in the right parietal lobe of her brain. The mass had been discovered during a hospitalization one month earlier, and she declined to have the biopsy at the time. Prior to that hospitalization she had bilateral lower extremity weakness (left worse than right), multiple falls over two weeks, and she wasn't able to walk at all the day before admission. A chest CT showed a 9-mm mildly spiculated (spiky) lung nodule, and the spicules were suggestive of cancer. She was readmitted to the hospital the day before her biopsy for a partial seizure that caused the left side of her head and neck and left arm to jerk for about 30 seconds.

Dr. Jackson performed the operation with Dr. Wilson assisting. Both doctors wore binocular loupe headsets for the delicate surgery. A U-shaped incision was made in the shaved, scrubbed scalp, and the flap of scalp was retracted. Two burr holes were made in the skull, and a craniotome was used to make a circular cut that connected the burr holes. The bone flap was removed to complete the craniotomy, and the membranous covering of the brain was carefully opened in a U shape.

"James, what are we opening?" Dr. Wilson said.

"The dura mater."

"Yes."

It was impressive to see the pulsating brain!

Dr. Jackson carefully resected part of the tumor, and the specimen was quickly taken to be examined by a pathologist. The pathologist called the OR intercom about 10 minutes later.

"Wayne, hi. This is Derek. The specimen is adequate, but I can't make a definitive diagnosis from the frozen section. This is a poorly differentiated neoplasm, probably a metastatic carcinoma,[1] but I need a permanent section to make a final diagnosis."

"Thanks, Wayne," Dr. Jackson said. "Have a good day."

"Thanks. You too."

Dr. Jackson carefully closed the dura mater with sutures and fibrin glue.

"James, why is it important to completely seal the dura?" Dr. Jackson said.

"So CSF won't leak."

"Yes."

The bone flap was replaced and secured with titanium plates and screws, and the scalp flap was closed.

The second case was a ventriculoperitoneal (VP) shunt removal for a 65-year-old female who had abdominal pain and a seroma (fluid collection) due to a malfunctioning shunt. Dr. Wilson performed the operation. A properly functioning VP shunt relieves pressure on the brain by draining excess CSF from a ventricle to the abdominal peritoneum for absorption. After we were done with the second case, I saw an inpatient with Dr. Jackson. The patient was a 73-year-old male with right wrist drop and 3-cm masses in the left parietal and right temporal lobes of his brain. He initially declined to have a biopsy, but he changed his mind the next day.

On Thursday morning the pathologist called Dr. Jackson in the clinic to let him know that the brain tumor in the 79-year-old female was a poorly differentiated metastatic carcinoma, and he requested a consult from another pathologist to try to determine the type of carcinoma. The consultant's diagnosis was received a week later: metastatic, poorly differentiated, non-small cell carcinoma.

The clinic was busier on Thursday. I saw patients with neck and back pain and radiculopathy. Most of them were obese, and some were smokers. A 58-year-old female weighed 375 pounds, and she had a history of bilateral lumbar discectomy for cauda equina syndrome, a rare condition that is a medical emergency and can cause incontinence and permanent paralysis of lower extremities if not treated quickly. An 89-year-old female was seen to review a follow-up MRI for a cerebellar intraparenchymal hemorrhage (bleed within brain tissue) that didn't require surgery. The bleed had been caused by poorly controlled HTN. The hematoma was resolving, and Dr. Jackson advised her to be compliant with her blood pressure medications. A 37-year-old male was seen to review a follow-up MRI after he had a burr hole and subdural drain placed in his skull to relieve pressure from a subdural hematoma. The hematoma was discovered with a CT scan in the ED, where he presented with a severe headache and vomiting three weeks after he struck his head on a rock in a river tubing accident.

Friday was a busier day in the OR. The first case was a stereotactic brain biopsy for a 63-year-old female with multiple masses in her cerebellum and cerebral hemispheres. The largest mass was 3.2 cm and located in the cerebellar vermis (median lobe that connects the two lateral lobes). The second largest mass was 1.2 cm and located in the right frontal cortex. Prior to hospitalization she had intractable vomiting, headache, and balance difficulty for two to three weeks, and she was running into things and leaning to a side. She had an extensive medical history, including non-small cell carcinoma of the lung. The cancer had been resected two months earlier, but she didn't receive any radiation or chemotherapy treatment.

Dr. Wilson performed the operation with Dr. Jackson assisting. The patient's head was placed in a frame, and the Brainlab neuronavigation equipment was calibrated to the MRI of her brain to map the brain with a three-dimensional coordinate system. A small U-shaped incision was made in the scalp just behind the hairline, and the flap was retracted. The Brainlab system was used to set a starting point and target, and a burr hole was created. The VarioGuide (biopsy needle holder) of the Brainlab system was calibrated and used to match the trajectory for the biopsy needle through the burr hole. After this was set up, corticectomy (removal of cerebral cortex) was performed with electrocautery, and the biopsy needle was advanced using neuronavigation image guidance. Once the target was reached, multiple biopsies were obtained. The pathologist told Dr. Wilson the tumor was a metastatic adenocarcinoma, a malignant tumor of epithelial cells with a glandular or glandlike pattern. The burr hole was covered with methyl methacrylate, a thermoplastic, and the scalp flap was closed.

The second case was an anterior cervical discectomy and fusion (ACDF) for a 54-year-old male who had an osteophyte complex at C5-6 (disc herniation with bone spurs around the margins of the vertebral endplates). Dr. Jackson performed the operation. A small incision was made in the right neck, and tissues were carefully dissected. The carotid pulse was palpated to ensure that dissection was done between the carotid sheath on one side and the trachea and esophagus on the other side. Tissues were retracted, and the disc level was confirmed by x-ray with a needle marker. The disc was carefully removed, and a small burr was used to remove the osteophytes and flatten the endplates. A bone graft was gently hammered in between the endplates and secured with a titanium plate and screws that went into the vertebrae above and below the graft. The wound was closed.

The third case was a L3–S1 decompression for a 52-year-old male with degenerative disc disease and an L4–5 disc bulge. Dr. Jackson performed laminectomies (removal of laminae) and removed osteophytes to relieve pressure from nerves. The fourth case was an open cranial temporal biopsy for the 73-year-old male with right wrist drop and 3-cm masses in the left parietal and right temporal lobes. The pathologist told Dr. Jackson the mass was a malignant tumor with epithelioid characteristics suggestive of a high-grade oligodendroglioma (a rare tumor that originates from oligodendroglia cells in the brain), but he needed a permanent section to make a final diagnosis. The consultant pathologist's diagnosis was received a week later: metastatic malignant melanoma.

On Friday evening Lynn and I drove to Hansen, Tennessee, to stay with friends for the weekend. On Saturday we had dinner with Dr. Anderson and Dr. Vaswani at Sachin's Taste of India. Dr. Anderson's wife and an Indian resident were also present. The resident was a thin, middle-aged man with short, black hair, and a red dot on his forehead like Dr. Vaswani. His face was long, angular, and Lynn and I agreed he looked creepy, especially since he never smiled and he barely talked — he mostly just stared while the rest of us conversed. I thought the dinner was delicious, but Lynn didn't like it as much. Not surprisingly, she also said Dr. Vaswani was weird. On Sunday we returned to Brighton.

On Monday of my second week I observed three more ACDFs and a T6–7 decompression for a 70-year-old male with masses in his lung, liver, and spine. The extradural spinal mass was causing vertebral bone destruction and compressing T6–7. The pathologist told Dr. Wilson the mass was a poorly differentiated neoplasm, probably a metastatic carcinoma, but he needed a permanent section to make a final diagnosis. The consultant pathologist's diagnosis was received a week later: metastatic non-small cell carcinoma.

On Tuesday I saw 19 patients in the clinic. All but two of them had spinal problems. Most of them were obese, and some were smokers. A 67-year-old female was seen to review a follow-up MRI for a cerebellar hemorrhage that didn't require surgery. The hemorrhage had been caused by Coumadin. An 80-year-old female was seen to review a follow-up MRI for a subdural hematoma that didn't require surgery. The hematoma had been caused by a fall with head trauma. Both patients were recovering well.

On Wednesday I observed a tricky L1–2 intradural tumor resection with microsurgical technique for a 44-year-old male who had low back pain, bilateral lower extremity pain, and a history of lumbar surgery 13 years earlier. Dr. Jackson performed the operation with Dr. Wilson assisting.

"You must be a curse," Dr. Jackson said to me.

"What do you mean?" I said.

"We've had more tumor cases since you've been with us than we've had in the last six months."

"I'm sorry."

"You should be," Dr. Wilson said.

"I'm glad I'm getting to see the cases."

"Well, I hope this is the last one for a while," Dr. Jackson said.

Electrode needles were placed in the patient's lower extremities for monitoring of possible nerve root injury. An incision was made in the upper lumbar region, and tissues were dissected down through the thoracolumbar fascia. The fascia was retracted, and the L1–2 disc was confirmed with a marker. T12, L1, and L2 laminectomies were performed. The ligamentum flavum was gently resected, and hemostatic agents were used to stop bleeding. The microscope was draped and moved into the operating field in sterile fashion. The dura was carefully opened and tacked up with sutures. Several nerve roots were in, around, and densely adhered to the tumor. They were dissected away using microsurgical technique, and nerve root monitoring showed no abnormal discharges. The tumor was then entered and debulked internally. Microsurgical technique was used to dissect the tumor away from the nerve roots without injuring the nerves, and the wound was closed.

I returned to the clinic on Thursday, and on Friday I only observed a lumbar discectomy. I returned home early, logged into the NBOME website, and thanked God for the great news that I PASSED the COMLEX Level 2-PE! I updated my electronic residency application with the result and transmitted it to the residency programs I interviewed for.

For the last two weeks of the rotation, I continued to see more patients in the clinic with spinal problems and older patients with subdural hematomas. I observed spine surgeries, but the tumor curse ended with the spinal tumor resection. During my third week I also wrestled with how to rank the psychiatry residency programs. I made a typewritten list of the programs to compare salaries, state income taxes, vacation time, and health insurance costs. I considered locations, prestige of institutions, facilities, and moonlighting opportunities. I also listened to my gut. Where could I see myself fitting in and being happy? Which programs had the happy residents? Which programs had the most Americans? Lynn and I wanted to move back to Hansen, but she agreed with my bad gut feeling about the UNT program. I also had a bad gut feeling about University of Kentucky, where two residents had scrambled into the program.

I logged into the National Resident Matching Program (NRMP) website a few days before the February 21 deadline and certified my Rank Order List:

1. Vanderbilt (only two weeks of vacation for first-year residents, but it was Vanderbilt, and Tennessee had no state income tax)
2. University of New Mexico (Western location, moonlighting opportunity, three weeks of vacation)
3. University of Utah (highest salary $47,625, great facilities, nearby ski resorts, three weeks of vacation)
4. University of Louisville (second highest salary $47,323, four weeks of vacation)
5. Southern Arizona University (new program, three weeks of vacation, and 10 holidays)
6. Wake Forest (lowest salary $43,000, highest state income tax 7%, two weeks of vacation for first-year residents, we didn't want to live in Winston-Salem)
7. University of Northeast Tennessee
8. University of Kentucky

During my last week in the clinic, I saw the 73-year-old male with right wrist drop and masses in his parietal and temporal lobes. Dr. Jackson referred him to an oncologist for treatment of metastatic melanoma, but the patient said he didn't know if he wanted to have chemotherapy because he had seen people suffer through chemotherapy and still die. On my last day in the clinic, I saw a 27-year-old female with Arnold-Chiari type 1 malformation, an uncommon condition characterized by herniation of the bottom tips of cerebellar tonsils through the foramen magnum (skull opening) and into the spinal canal. At the end of the day, I thanked Drs. Jackson and Wilson for the experience, and Dr. Jackson gave me a glowing evaluation.

Endnotes

1. A carcinoma is a malignant neoplasm (tumor) that develops from epithelial cells that cover outer and inner surfaces of the body.

Chapter 21

The Final Stretch!

I really enjoyed my required two-month family medicine rotation with Dr. Coleman at the beginning of my third year, so I did an additional election rotation with him in March. This was my final rotation, and it was hard to believe I was near the end of my fourth and final, glorious year of medical school! I had survived a rotation with a borderline ob-gyn, who nearly failed me, and my second attempt at the dreaded COMLEX Level 2-PE. I saw the best and worst in humanity and even patients who have seen glimpses of heaven and hell. The experience was remarkable. Cherry trees and flowers were starting to bloom, grass was turning greener, and people started mowing their lawns.

"I know you asked to do another rotation with me because you knew it would be easy," Dr. Coleman said on my first day.

I smiled. "I enjoyed my rotation with you. I saw lots of interesting cases."

"Don't tell me you don't have any senioritis. I know I did in my fourth year."

"I may have a touch of the senioritis. Now I'm just waiting for Match Day."

"When is that?"

"March nineteenth."

"What's your top pick?"

"Vanderbilt, but I probably won't match there."

"Well, congratulations on getting an interview at Vanderbilt!"

"Thanks. I also interviewed at Wake Forest, but I ranked them toward the bottom of the list. Their salary's the lowest, state income tax is the highest, I'd only get two weeks of vacation in my first year, and my wife and I don't want to live in Winston-Salem."

"Wake Forest has the lowest salary? That's surprising for a school that's loaded. What's your second pick?"

"University of New Mexico."

"Well, that's a long way from Vanderbilt!"

"Yeah. I lived in Colorado for a few years, and I love the West. I didn't get an interview in Colorado, but I interviewed in New Mexico, Utah, and Arizona."

"Where else did you interview?"

"UofL, UK, UNT."

"So you could end up anywhere!"

"Yeah."

"Well, enjoy this rotation while you can 'cause you'll be a slave in a few months. Residents are the cheapest doctors in the country. They'll wear you out with the crazies."

"Thanks for the encouragement."

"You're welcome!" He smiled brightly and slapped me on the shoulder.

I saw more interesting cases with Dr. Coleman while his partner, Dr. Hunt, enjoyed having a cute, blonde, third-year medical student with him. On Friday, March 19, I was on pins and needles as I waited until 1 p.m. to find out where Lynn and I would be spending the next four years. When the time came, I anxiously logged into the NRMP website in Dr. Coleman's office, and my heart sank.

"I'm going to Arizona," I said.

"Arizona," Dr. Coleman said. "How did you rank them?"

"Fifth. I didn't expect to match that far down my list."

"Well, at least you didn't have to scramble. That would be hell."

"True. This is a new program. That's why I ranked them lower. But they offer the most vacation time."

"That's cool."

"Yeah. I can't believe I'm going to Arizona."

A couple of days later, Dr. Anderson sent me a text message, saying he was sorry I didn't match with the UNT program. I replied, thanking him again, and said I was headed west. At the end of my last rotation of medical school, I thanked Dr. Coleman for the experience, and he wished me well.

"Don't let the crazies get to you," he said with a bright smile.

Since I hadn't taken extra time off from my rotations to study for my COMLEX exams, I had the month of April off! Lynn happily resigned from her bank teller job at the end of March. I had been approved for a physician home loan offered to fourth-year-medical students, so we flew to Arizona for a week and looked at 10 houses in Tucson and Dillon, where the residency was based. Our top pick was a 1,700-square foot ranch house with three bedrooms in Dillon. The house was only four years old, and it was a foreclosure from the aftermath of the 2008 mortgage crisis. Ceiling fans had been removed, but the house was otherwise in fine shape. By the end of the week, the bank owner accepted our offer of $137,000, and our monthly mortgage payments would only be $689!

After we returned from Arizona, we visited our families in North Carolina, West Tennessee, and Western Kentucky. On May 7 our families came to Brighton: my father, Aunt Martha and her husband, my brother and his wife, Lynn's parents, sister, and niece. My father and Lynn's parents attended my graduation dinner with us. My stepmother didn't come because she was on a Mediterranean cruise with her two sisters and a niece.

After dinner Lynn and I met our good friends Chris and Jamie Devlin at a dumpy motel, where they were having drinks with their families. The Devlins were an interesting couple. Like Lynn and me, they met at an upscale restaurant where they worked together. Chris was overweight, handsome, with brown hair and a goatee, and he was a sharp dresser. He looked like Aidan Gillen, the Irish actor best known for portraying Petyr "Littlefinger" Baelish in the HBO series *Game of Thrones*. Chris was a meat eater and loudmouthed Republican, who often cursed and joked, which was understandable, considering that he was the eleventh child of a Catholic family. Jamie was a petite, cute, makeup-averse hippie with long, dirty blonde hair. She was a vegetarian, a gentle Democrat, and an attorney, who did nonprofit work and served indigent clients. She was an only child, and she hadn't cared for religion since her father had been murdered years earlier. Chris didn't care for church either. Lynn and I were Republicans, and Jamie didn't mind having civilized conversations about politics with three Republicans in the room. None of us ever became upset or angry when we talked about politics.

Jamie handed Lynn a Blue Moon beer, and Chris poured too much cheap vodka and some cranberry juice into a plastic cup for me. The Devlins were jovial.

"I can't believe we've made it!" Chris said, smiling brightly. "I can't believe we're gonna be fucking doctors, man!"

"Me either!" I said. "I had to go back to Conshofucken, Pennsylvania, to retake the damn COMLEX PE."

"I did too!"

"Really!"

"Yes."

"How did *that* happen? You're in the top 10 percent of the class."

"Our school should have trained us for that fucking exam. Other schools do."

"I know. I heard too many people in our class failed it, and they're planning to start a course for it next year."

"That exam was hell, man. I had panic attacks and felt like I was running around like a fucking chicken with its head cut off."

"Me too! I panicked the first time, so I took a Xanax the night before I took it the second time."

"I even had nightmares about it."

"Really?"

"Yeah. Well, here's to us never having to go back to Conshofucken, Pennsylvania!" Chris happily raised his drink.

"Amen to that!"

We clinked our plastic cups and took a drink. I only had a couple of vodka cranberries with Chris, but I had some bourbon with my brother after we returned to our apartment. And, of course, I regretted it the next morning. I was hungover on May 8, my graduation day! I took ibuprofen, Benadryl, drank water, and arrived at the Brighton College auditorium backstage at 8 a.m. for a photograph with my 73 classmates. Everyone was happy, smiling, conversing, except Chris didn't look so good.

"How are you feeling?" I said.

"Like shit," Chris said. "How are you?"

"Same. I've got a bad headache. I feel a little dizzy and nauseous, and ibuprofen and Benadryl haven't helped. I've been drinking water."

"I need to do that too."

After I smiled for the camera, our class walked into the auditorium, and I was blindsided by suddenly feeling tearful. As I struggled to hold back the tears, I thought about my dear, deceased mother, and I wished she were there. My father was a communication professor with a Ph.D., so he was my guest hooder. After I received my very expensive D.O. diploma, and I shook half a dozen hands, including the hand of Senator Mitch McConnell, my father proudly placed the green hood on me.

After graduation Lynn and I enjoyed a weeklong Lake Tahoe vacation with the Devlins. Jamie's mother had a condo timeshare at a ski resort there, so we only had to pay for our flights and rental car. Her mother's house was close to the Cincinnati airport, so we all stayed with her the night before our morning flight. Chris and I were hungover again on our departure day because we had too much to drink the night before. We took ibuprofen and Benadryl and slept our headaches away on the plane. May wasn't an ideal month to vacation at Lake Tahoe. It was mud season, the time between ski resort closures and summer activities. Temperatures ranged from the upper 20s to low 60s, and a few inches of snow fell almost every day. The fresh snow quickly melted away, but hiking trails were still covered with snowpack. The area was like a ghost town, which was kind of cool.

Chris and I continued to drink too much during the week, but we didn't have any more bad hangovers. We cooked meals in our condo, had delicious pizza and beer at the nearby Stateline Brewery, and dinner at a Thai restaurant. In the evenings we soaked in an outdoor hot tub that was on a top-floor balcony at the end of the hall. The balcony offered a great view of Lake Tahoe and the jagged, snowy Sierra Nevada Mountains in the distance.

We drove all the way around Lake Tahoe, which is bisected by the California/Nevada state line. According to the Most Beautiful Drive in America brochure, the trip is a "72-mile scenic journey unlike any in the world. At 22 miles long and 12 miles wide, Lake Tahoe is North America's largest alpine lake. The lake contains enough water to cover the entire state of California to a depth of 14 inches. The water is 99 percent pure, and a white dinner plate can be seen to a depth of 70 feet." The drive was impressive. The water was incredibly clear, blue, and green, and the lake was surrounded by white mountains. We made many stops along our drive to enjoy the scenery and take photos. Our favorite stops were Emerald Bay Lookout on the southwest side of the lake in California and Sand Harbor on the northeast side of the lake in Nevada. The Emerald Bay Lookout offered a spectacular overlook of the bay, which was "one of the most photographed places in the world." We had a picnic lunch in the cedars and Jeffrey pines of Sand Harbor, which had sandy beaches meeting boulder-strewn shoreline. After lunch we explored the area and shed our coats as the sun warmed the cold air. We took lots of photos and strolled along a boardwalk.

After Lynn and I returned from our awesome Lake Tahoe vacation, we packed up a 22-foot, yellow Penske truck with the help of four third-year medical students. A 16-foot truck would have been big enough for our meager belongings, but the larger truck had more power to tow Lynn's Toyota Camry. I was very nervous when I first drove it, towing a car dolly, to our apartment. I couldn't believe anyone was allowed to drive the big trucks without any training. Chad Dudley was one of the students who helped us. He and his wife, Katherine, made us a delicious, hot dinner, and they insisted that we sleep in their bed because our bed was packed up. We expressed our heartfelt gratitude. We were exhausted, and we slept well. In the morning I started the clattering diesel engine, Lynn started my Volvo sedan, and we began our 1,983-mile journey to our next adventure!

Epilogue

In April 2016, Eric C. Conn, the "Mr. Social Security" attorney, and his coconspirators were indicted for defrauding the Social Security Administration of $550 million. Conn had become a multimillionaire by representing more disability cases than any other law firm in Kentucky. He had used aggressive advertising and paid a family physician, a psychiatrist, and two judges to rubber-stamp applications. He pleaded guilty in March 2017 and agreed to testify against others, but in June he fled from the FBI. He had been under house arrest when he cut off his ankle monitor one month before his sentencing hearing. He was arrested in December 2017 in Honduras, and at age 57 he was sentenced to a total of 27 years in prison.

In 2019 Purdue Pharma filed for bankruptcy as the company and its owners, the Sackler family, faced 3,000 lawsuits (including suits from 48 states) for misleading the public on OxyContin's risk of addiction. In March 2022 Purdue reached a nationwide settlement over its role in the opioid crisis. The company could pay more than $10 billion over time, with $6 billion coming from the Sacklers' $13 billion fortune. The Sacklers relinquished control of Purdue so the company could be reformed as a trust to fight the opioid epidemic.

According to a Sept. 25, 2018, NBC News article, Katherine Hoover, M.D., was extremely busy when she worked for Mountain Medical Care Center, the notorious pill mill in Williamson, West Virginia. From December 2002 to January 2010, Dr. Hoover wrote 335,130 opioid prescriptions—a rate of 130 per day if she worked seven days a week—more than any other doctor in the state, even though Williamson only had 3,000 residents. In 2020 West Virginia had the nation's highest rate of opioid overdose deaths.

According to undercover federal investigators, hundreds of customers lined up outside Mountain Medical every day, starting at 6 a.m., and some of them lived hours away. New customers paid $450 in cash to see a doctor and get a prescription, and returning customers paid $150 to a receptionist, who handed out new prescriptions after asking a cursory question or two about their health. In 2009 the clinic took in more than $4.6 million in cash. According to the Mingo County prosecuting attorney, people called the tiny town "Pilliamson."

On March 2, 2010, federal investigators ended a two-year undercover probe by raiding the clinic and shutting it down. Amazingly, Dr. Hoover was never charged with a crime, and the reason remains a mystery. The U.S. attorney's office in Charleston and the former federal prosecutor in charge of the case, Booth Goodwin, didn't respond to NBC News calls for comment on why they didn't pursue criminal charges against Dr. Hoover. Four days after the feds raided Mountain Medical, Hoover fled to the Bahamas, where she and her husband said they owned the 700-acre Little Ragged Island. Her suspended medical license was revoked in May 2010 for a different reason. She failed to make a periodic appearance before the Board of Medicine, which was a requirement since she was accused of asking a 17-year-old patient if she or any of her friends would have sex with her teenage sons in 1995.

In 2012 William Ryckman, M.D., who also worked in the clinic, was convicted of selling prescriptions to people he never examined. He was sentenced to six months in prison, and $413,050.89 was confiscated from a Mountain Medical account that was listed in his name. He was reluctant to talk to NBC News about Dr. Hoover, but he did say she wrote many opioid prescriptions for patients she never saw. "She was the softest person," he said. "Any time I tried to get people off medication, they would go to her, and she would just keep increasing people's medication." In 2013 Myra Sue Miller, the office manager, pleaded guilty to misusing Dr. Ryckman's DEA number, and she was sentenced to six months in prison. She declined to discuss Dr. Hoover through her attorney. As part of her plea agreement, she turned over two buildings worth more than $600,000 to the government, and more than $475,823 in cash was confiscated from her Williamson home.

In 2011 ob-gyn Lindsey Border, M.D., lost her BMC privileges after she threw another tantrum in the OR and hit a nurse while she was on probation for her behavior.

In 2011 Hiral Vaswani, M.D., program director of the UNT psychiatry residency, was forced to resign after the American Council for Graduate Medical Education received several anonymous complaints, alleging that he "greatly favors residents of Indian descent," meets with a select group of residents at his house at night to discuss the program and other residents, that the select group had access to other residents' personal information and test scores, and that there is "great discrimination regarding duty assignments, distribution of rotations, and work load among residents." The complaints also alleged that the resident work schedule was being made by first- and second-year Indian residents. My bad gut feeling about UNT was right!

In 2012 psychiatrist Robert Damron, M.D., had his medical license revoked for allegedly having sex with several male patients, including a 16-year-old. He accepted a plea agreement on the day his trial was to begin. He was sentenced to six months in jail, 18 months of probation, and he would be on a sex offender registry for life.

In 2014 James Banks, D.O., graduated from the Southern Arizona University psychiatry residency and started a very challenging psychiatrist job at the Arizona State Prison Complex, Tucson, where 5,000 inmates were incarcerated.

Acknowledgements

Thank you to my wife, Kelly, for being supportive of this writing endeavor, my sister, Carrie, for being my first editor, and my father, Marcus, for correcting my English when I was a child.

James Champion is a psychiatrist practicing in Appalachia. He supervises psychiatry residents, teaches medical students, and collaborates with nurse practitioners. He has a D.O. degree from an Appalachian medical school. This is his first book.

ROUNDFIRE
BOOKS

FICTION

Historical fiction that lives

Put simply, we publish great stories. Whether it's literary or popular, a gentle tale or a pulsating thriller, the connecting theme in all Roundfire fiction titles is that once you pick them up you won't want to put them down.

If you have enjoyed this book, why not tell other readers by posting a review on your preferred book site.

Recent bestsellers from Roundfire are:

The Bookseller's Sonnets
Andi Rosenthal

The Bookseller's Sonnets intertwines three love stories with a tale of religious identity and mystery spanning five hundred years and three countries.

Paperback: 978-1-84694-342-3 ebook: 978-184694-626-4

Birds of the Nile
An Egyptian Adventure

N.E. David

Ex-diplomat Michael Blake wanted a quiet birding trip up the Nile – he wasn't expecting a revolution.

Paperback: 978-1-78279-158-4 ebook: 978-1-78279-157-7

Blood Profit$
The Lithium Conspiracy

J. Victor Tomaszek, James N. Patrick, Sr.

The blood of the many for the profits of the few. . . *Blood Profit$* will take you into the cigar-smoke-filled room where American policy and laws are really made.

Paperback: 978-1-78279-483-7 ebook: 978-1-78279-277-2

The Burden
A Family Saga

N.E. David

Frank will do anything to keep his mother and father apart. But he's carrying baggage – and it might just weigh him down. .

Paperback: 978-1-78279-936-8 ebook: 978-1-78279-937-5

The Cause
Roderick Vincent
The second American Revolution will be a fire lit from an internal spark.
Paperback: 978-1-78279-763-0 ebook: 978-1-78279-762-3

Don't Drink and Fly
The Story of Bernice O'Hanlon: Part One
Cathie Devitt
Bernice is a witch living in Glasgow. She loses her way in her life and wanders off the beaten track looking for the garden of enlightenment.
Paperback: 978-1-78279-016-7 ebook: 978-1-78279-015-0

Gag
Melissa Unger
One rainy afternoon in a Brooklyn diner, Peter Howland punctures an egg with his fork. Repulsed, Peter pushes the plate away and never eats again.
Paperback: 978-1-78279-564-3 ebook: 978-1-78279-563-6

The Master Yeshua
The Undiscovered Gospel of Joseph
Joyce Luck
Jesus is not who you think he is. The year is 75 CE. Joseph ben Jude is frail and ailing, but he has a prophecy to fulfil . . .
Paperback: 978-1-78279-974-0 ebook: 978-1-78279-975-7

On the Far Side, There's a Boy
Paula Coston
Martine Haslett, a thirty-something 1980s woman, plays hard on the fringes of the London drag club scene until one night which prompts her to sign up to a charity. She writes to a young Sri Lankan boy, with consequences far and long.
Paperback: 978-1-78279-574-2 ebook: 978-1-78279-573-5

Tuareg
Alberto Vazquez-Figueroa
With over 5 million copies sold worldwide, *Tuareg* is a classic adventure story from best-selling author Alberto Vazquez-Figueroa, about honour, revenge and a clash of cultures.
Paperback: 978-1-84694-192-4

Readers of ebooks can buy or view any of these bestsellers by clicking on the live link in the title. Most titles are published in paperback and as an ebook. Paperbacks are available in traditional bookshops. Both print and ebook formats are available online.

Find more titles and sign up to our readers' newslett er at
http://www.johnhuntpublishing.com/fiction

Follow us on Facebook at https://www.facebook.com/
JHPfiction and Twitter at https://twitter.com/JHPFiction